THE
24/7
BODY

Matt Morsia (MattDoesFitness) is the UK's No. 1 Fitness Vlogger, with over 240 million views on YouTube. A former athlete, PE teacher and personal trainer, he is known for his funny, honest and informative fitness advice and videos, and for his hilarious son Luca and wife Sarah. He has attempted some of the world's hardest, most extreme and most unusual training and diet regiments. From the Rock's workout to the Navy Seals fitness test, he shares what works, and what doesn't. Drawing on cutting-edge sports and nutritional science, Matt dispels the myths, fad diets and workouts, to provide viewers with incredible results that last.

T0010651

THE 24/7 BODY

MATT MORSIA

PENGUIN BOOKS

PENGUIN BOOKS

UK | USA | Canada | Ireland | Australia
India | New Zealand | South Africa

Penguin Books is part of the Penguin Random House group of companies
whose addresses can be found at global.penguinrandomhouse.com

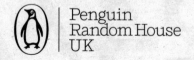

First published by Century in 2020
Published in Penguin Books in 2021
001

Copyright © Matt Does Fitness Ltd

The moral right of the author has been asserted

Typeset by Jouve (UK), Milton Keynes

Printed and bound in Great Britain by Clays Ltd, Elcograf S.p.A.

The authorised representative in the EEA is Penguin Random House Ireland,
Morrison Chambers, 32 Nassau Street, Dublin D02 YH68

A CIP catalogue record for this book is available from the British Library

ISBN: 978–1–787–46732–3

www.greenpenguin.co.uk

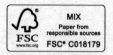

Note to readers: This book is based on my personal experiences and learning and has been compiled as general guidance on the specific subjects approached, and I hope you may find some of my approaches useful. I'm not a nutritionist or a medical professional and this book is not a substitute for professional nutritional, medical or healthcare advice. If you have a mental health issue, an eating disorder, or are considering starting a diet, I'd strongly advise that you go and see a specialist for professional advice immediately, as you may require medical help. In terms of changes in nutrition, you should first talk to a doctor or registered dietician. Please consult your GP before changing, stopping or starting any medical treatment.

For Sairs, Luca and the new arrival

CONTENTS

INTRODUCTION

I can't believe they're letting me write a book. Like, an actual book. This is ridiculous. My GCSE English teacher is going to absolutely kick off. It probably won't even be that good to be honest. I can barely speak, let alone write. In fact, why did you even buy it? What were you thinking?! That was a joke. It's probably going to be the best thing anyone's ever written. Nice one for buying it, much appreciated. Anyway, now that the awkward first paragraph is pretty much sorted, let me explain why I wanted to write this. Oh, and if at any point I come across as a massive narcissist, I apologise. I'm not actually a massive narcissist. I don't think I am anyway. It's just really hard to write a book, some of which is about yourself without sounding like a bit of a dick.

So, as a former PE teacher, athlete, personal trainer and now one of the biggest fitness YouTubers in the world (aka a weirdo who gets paid to film themselves doing stuff), the most common question I get from followers and even people in the street is, 'How do I get a body like yours?' (great start with the whole not coming across as a massive narcissist thing). People will almost whisper it, as if I'm going to usher them into a dark alleyway and reveal some kind of mystical secret. I think they're expecting to be told that they need to drink 23ml of maple syrup eight times a day while reading the complete works of Shakespeare to their auntie's hamster. Or something equally ridiculous. Other times they want me to outline a protocol of supplements, with the inference that I must be taking steroids or other drugs, because having a decent physique without chemicals is now seen by most as almost impossible.

People are always looking for some elusive quick fix, and I feel like a constant source of disappointment when I offer up my fairly simple and not particularly sexy advice. The truth is that, despite everything you have been told, there is no secret. No magic supplement or superfood; no esoteric or excessive routine that in a short space of time and with minimal effort is going to transform your body. Unfortunately, that's not how it works, and even if you are able to follow a crash diet and lose loads of weight in the space of a few weeks, I guarantee you will eventually put it all back on and then some.

This is one of the reasons why I've held off from writing a book about fitness and the body for so long – because, despite what most people on social media and in the fitness industry would have you believe, the most effective methods of losing fat, building muscle or 'toning up' are actually very simple. So simple, in fact, that after reading this book you'll be capable of doing them yourself. Just wait and see.

Now don't get me wrong, social media *can* be awesome. But as someone who has a degree in Sports Therapy and Exercise Physiology and has competed internationally in both athletics and powerlifting (with over fifteen years' experience as a sports coach and personal trainer), I find the abundance of absolute shite being promoted by many 'fitness influencers' infuriating. That noise only adds to the already crazy confusion of messages that we have been fed about the body from the fitness and diet industries, as well as the conflicting information that the government and even doctors have given us over the years. It is extremely frustrating to watch all of this play out, knowing that there are millions of people following terrible advice and, as a result, not managing to improve their health, fitness or body composition.

This book is my attempt to shatter all of those myths and clear up this wealth of misinformation. Eating McDonald's doesn't make you fat. Eating a salad won't make you skinny.

Doing sit-ups won't get rid of your belly fat and losing loads of weight in a couple of weeks isn't a good thing. I could go on but hopefully you get the point. So many of the things we've been brought up to believe are completely false and this is one of the major reasons why people struggle to change their bodies and achieve their fitness goals.

Just to be clear here – I'm not going to change the way you look and feel in two weeks. If that's what you're after then put the book down and go and try a few more of the 'cutting edge' fat loss methods you discovered in *Heat* magazine. Then, once you've realised that they don't actually work in the long run, come back and read this book. I don't want to sound overly dramatic, and I'm not necessarily going for the 'tough love' approach, because I have a lot of empathy for people struggling with diet and body shape, but if you're not ready to accept that genuine change comes from a more permanent reframing of your habits and behaviour, then you're not ready for this book. The reason it's called *The 24/7 Body* is because finding an equilibrium and happiness in your body isn't something you can just dabble in. It's not a temporary state. It has to become a way of life. Forever.

Now, before you sprint in the other direction, I'm not in any way suggesting that you have to turn into some kind of monk to have a great body and be healthy and happy. I am living proof of that. If you've watched any of my YouTube videos, you'll know that I frequently eat 'crappy' food – I always have, and honestly, it's why I will never compete in bodybuilding or embark on any career that requires me to completely eradicate junk food from my diet. Krispy Kremes and Pizza Hut are *way* too important to me to let that happen. I truly believe that any diet that says you can't have doughnuts, pizza or chocolate is doomed to failure. And I actually think it's dangerous to label any particular food as 'bad' or tell people they should avoid it at all costs, because, as well as being untrue, this is often a one-way ticket to an eating disorder.

Now obviously you can't eat crap all day every day and expect to build the body of your dreams. But at the same time, eating junk food every now and again won't stop you from achieving your goals. Ultimately it comes down to moderation. It might be the most boring word in the dictionary, but with a solid understanding of the power of moderation, you can transform its meaning from boring to liberating. Moderation means that you can eat what you want (within reason) while keeping fit and healthy. You don't even have to think of it as 'falling off the wagon', because it's part of the wagon. It *is* the wagon. *You* are the wagon. (Sorry, that's way too many wagons for one paragraph.) Applying words like 'cheating' or 'sinning' to the food you eat is ridiculous. I'd argue that it's these kinds of words that have ruined our understanding of balanced eating and cause a lot of emotional issues when it comes to our eating patterns.

I also didn't want this book to be yet another cheesy manual that sounds nothing like the author on the front cover. We've all read those sorts of books and felt massively disappointed, and it would be my literal nightmare to have my name attached to anything like that. I am hugely appreciative to you for picking up this book and for giving it a go. I am also hugely appreciative of my audience online for supporting me. It's really important to me that this isn't just another fitness book churned out to make some money. I have over fifteen years of experience in this field and I've dedicated a huge amount of time to research, consulting hundreds of studies and pieces of academic and scientific literature. Anecdotal evidence can be extremely useful, but I want you to know that I won't tell you something unless I know it to be true and have evidence to support it.

On top of that I also wanted to give you an insight into some of the challenges and difficulties I've personally been through when it comes to pushing my own body to change – for both good and bad. It's still a taboo to talk about some of the issues I'll address, particularly when it comes to eating disorders, but I know from my experience with thousands of clients that these kinds of issues are massively prevalent. Being open with this kind of thing can be a challenge, but there will be people reading this book going through something similar and I want you to know that you are not alone. I also think it's really important to understand that the way someone looks isn't always a good indication of their overall health (or knowledge) – something that's worth remembering when we're scrolling through social media.

When it comes to training and exercise, this book won't offer a one-size-fits-all plan, because that would be selling you another lie. Coming up with a generic programme which anyone can follow goes against pretty much everything I believe in and, more importantly, it doesn't work. There's no way you can create a plan that is optimal for an overweight sixty-year-old woman and an underweight twenty-year-old man. Anyone who tells you otherwise is mugging you off. If I have 100 different clients, they will follow 100 different plans. In terms of diet, even the concept of a 'plan' itself is flawed. That is, it suggests something that will tide you over for six or eight weeks and then it's over. You can just go back to your old life. And that is exactly what is wrong with the messages that we are fed by the fitness and diet industries. Instead, I want to give *you* the knowledge and the skills to empower *yourself* to make permanent changes to your life. It sounds ridiculously cheesy but it's true. By understanding the concept of energy balance (energy meaning the calories in food – I'm not talking about star signs) and basic physiology – how your body works and reacts to exercise – you won't need to be constantly flicking through the pages of this or any other book. It's about understanding how to live your life in a more healthy, sustainable and happy way – and how to maintain that forever.

Right, introduction done. Sick. Let's get stuck in to the good stuff. I really hope you love this book by the way – I genuinely believe it will help a lot of people. Also, if you have any questions or want to ask me about anything you've read, you know where to find me.

(I'm talking about YouTube or Instagram by the way. Don't come to my house. That would be weird.)

Matt

CHAPTER ONE

I HAVE AN EATING DISORDER

Seeing as you're literally reading my book, I feel that I should probably take this opportunity to tell you a bit about myself, just so you know I'm not an absolute serial killer. In fairness, if I was a serial killer I probably wouldn't tell you about it due to the whole prison thing, so I guess you're just going to have to take my word for it. I suppose my first task is to make you trust me on a level that goes beyond just the way I look, and the best way to do that is to give you a bit more of an idea of who I am and the journey I've been on to get here. (On a side note, when someone uses the word journey to describe anything other than an actual journey – like driving to Aldi for example – it makes me want to punch them in the face, but as I'm writing an actual book I'm going to have to write dorky stuff like that from time to time. Soz about that.)

Anyway, I think that in order to show you what I've learnt, how it's helped me and how it could help you too, I should give you a bit of my backstory. Now, unless you're an absolute superfan (aka a weirdo), you might not be waiting with bated breath for my entire life story, but don't worry – nearly everything I'm going to mention here will lead back to specific learnings which will help to anchor my fitness and nutrition philosophies. Getting to know what I've put my body (and stomach) through will hopefully provide some useful context for all of the ideas I'm about to share with you, because I am my best case study.

So, let's start from the very beginning. I have always been a sporty person. As a kid I was massively active, and my elder sister and I would spend our evenings playing with the other kids on our road until we were dragged in for dinner. When I say playing, I mean participating in a series of highly competitive races against one another, whereby anything went – bikes, rollerblades, skateboards – it was an absolute free for all. And when I say participating, I mean desperately trying to win every single race as if our lives depended on it. Actually, on reflection, that was probably just me. You see, for as long as I can remember, I've always been desperate to be the best at everything I do, whether it was winning a race with my mates, or eating my cereal first. Literally *anything* I was involved in became a competition.

Once my younger brother (I have two, but the nearest one in age to me) was old enough to get involved, he became my new 'training partner' and we'd do everything together. I remember walking to the nearest park every day after school to play football with the older kids, and even at that age desperately wanting to improve and being obsessed by the process of getting better at stuff. By the time I was eleven (my family had moved down from London to Kent at this point and I was just starting my third stint at a new primary school), I was already the quickest in my school year and would regularly win the weekly bicep showdown. In hindsight, this was fairly weird, but it essentially involved a few of the bigger/stronger boys comparing the size of their biceps and the winner of the contest being decided by the nearest dinner lady. It has to be said that, at the time, I took a huge amount of pride in this title. Anyway, that year I started playing for the school football team and I totally fell in love with it – my whole family are massive Arsenal fans – devoting every spare minute to playing football and getting better at it. I progressed pretty quickly as a footballer and an athlete, and after getting into the local grammar school, which was really sports-orientated, I made a big jump and began playing for the county.

Although I'd say I took football seriously, I think, like a lot of teenagers, I had some serious failings when it came to my motivation. At the time, I loved to stay within my comfort zone and could be easily intimidated by anything outside of that. I had all my mates around me at school and in my club and I just didn't ever feel up to pushing myself beyond that and meeting new people. Some of that was laziness, but I do think a lot of kids hold themselves back from opportunities because they lack the confidence to take the next step.

By the time I reached fifteen, I'd also started doing athletics. It all began with an inter-house tournament where they were short on people and I ended up being drafted in to do the long and triple jumps. I was quick, but I'd never really jumped before, so I was surprised when during that first competition, I broke the school triple jump record which had stood for over twenty years. It was a bit of wake-up call really, and I remember everyone saying it was a big deal, but I still considered myself a footballer and had big aspirations to play professionally.

It was while I was at sixth form that my focus began to transition to athletics. I was still playing football, but as I started training for triple jump at the local athletics stadium in Ashford, I was picked up by a coach who helped me put together my first proper training plan. I actually remember rushing home to tell my parents that I'd given my phone number to an old man I'd met at the track and then being confused when they weren't immediately delighted for me.

At the same time, I was on a run of football-related injuries, which culminated in an ankle sprain brought about by a game we used to play at school. It essentially involved seeing who could jump (and land) from the highest step, and being the pathologically competitive individual that I was, I decided it was a good idea to jump an entire flight of stairs – which inevitably ended badly. Unfortunately, I was due to travel to the US on the school football tour a few weeks later and so ended up playing most of the games using only my weaker but non-injured left foot. This was the final straw for me. I can remember being constantly frustrated that I was never fully fit and it got to the point where I realised I was going to have to choose between athletics and football, and in the the end triple jump won.

What I liked most about athletics (aside from the fact that I was quite good at it) was that the outcome was almost entirely dependent on me. If I trained hard I would do better; if I didn't, I wouldn't improve. I can remember sometimes getting impatient with football, because we'd often lose, even if I'd played really well. I loved my mates, but we weren't a brilliant team. I'm not saying that I don't like the camaraderie of team sports, because I really do, but there's something deeply satisfying about knowing that what you put in as an individual, you'll get back. When I decide to do something, I'll typically do it wholeheartedly and, if it's sport-related, I'll train as much as I need to get better. If I'm not getting better, or at least in a position to control whether or not I *can* get better, I'm not interested. I like knowing that I'm in control of the outcome and I love being able to see that progression.

I think lots of the successes I've had in both my sporting and subsequent careers have stemmed from my abnormal obsession with tracking progress. I'm basically a sporty Rainman. Whether it's seeing that progress in a numerical sense – watching your results get better and better – or seeing growth happen physically, it has always been a huge driver for me. As kids, my younger brother and I would play the *Championship Manager* computer game for hours on end. During the school holidays, it wasn't uncommon for us to put in a twelve-hour shift, and I loved working on a long-term strategy and seeing my team grow and get promoted. It was exactly the same with athletics, and that's one of the things that made it perfect for me. I had training diaries for absolutely everything and I wrote down every single tiny detail, whether it was how far I jumped, how fast I ran or how much I lifted. I would constantly monitor and analyse my progress, making sure I was moving forward, doing more and getting bigger and better. I still get a huge amount of satisfaction and gratification from seeing my progress now and I think that really links to what I'm doing on social media too, where there is so much data for me to look at and work out ways to improve. Wanting to keep tabs on things is definitely part of my personality.

Weirdly, this part of my psyche was generally limited to things of a sporting nature and I didn't really apply any of that attitude to school. By all accounts, I was a pretty smart kid, but I was just not fussed with academics. I suppose the big problem was that I knew from a really young age that I wanted to do something physical in my future, so the rest of it all felt like a waste of time. This didn't mean I didn't work really hard at school. When it came to sport, I was so driven – I was constantly training, and I performed really well in the sporting arena – but we still don't really value that in the same way as we would a straight A student, at least in this country. If sports were held in higher esteem in schools and prioritised in the same way as, say, maths or English, it could be transformative for millions of children – especially if there was also adequate education around nutrition and fitness.

After school, I got a place on a Sports Therapy course at the University of Kent, which was about an hour's drive from home. I lived about fifteen minutes from the athletics track, so this meant that I could train every day, though in hindsight it also meant that I missed out on a lot of the non-academic side of uni. It was always, 'I've got to go home,' or 'I'm training, so I can't make it,' but in my head I was going to be an Olympic triple jumper, so nothing else really mattered. Everything I did was concentrated on reaching that goal. The training I was doing at the time was a mix of strength and conditioning work and technique-focused jumping drills. There was a lot of sprinting but also a good amount of weightlifting, and this was the first time I was properly exposed to resistance training. I started squatting, bench pressing and performing the Olympic lifts, but would also throw in some bodybuilding training after my sessions, which wasn't really compatible with triple jumping, because the optimal physique for a jumper is very slim with a low body weight. There certainly isn't any room to carry upper body mass, and every extra pound of muscle in that area can be detrimental to your performance.

Although this was my first structured experience of weight training, I had been dabbling in it since the age of fourteen when my uncle gave me a small set of dumbbells. I had no idea what I was doing with them to be fair, but that didn't stop me sitting at home every night doing arm curls in my bedroom like an absolute creep. After a few months I became noticeably bigger, and I liked the feeling of growing physically, and definitely enjoyed looking more muscular. I was really into action films and was also a huge WWE fan. The Rock was my absolute hero – I still devote entire

YouTube videos to him even now – I had his posters all over my walls and I even saw him at a WWE event in London and forced my dad to buy me one of his signature T-shirts. This is pretty embarrassing to admit, but I remember stitching the sleeves of it to make them tighter so they would cling to my biceps. Looking back, it's clear that even as a fourteen-year-old boy, I was very aware of my body image and wanted to improve it. We know now that body image issues start much earlier than previous generations realised, and as a mid-teen it was something that was definitely on my mind.

Behind my coach's back, either in the gym or at home, I was lifting heavier and heavier weights. I thought I knew what I was doing, but I was pretty clueless and it was starting to become counter-productive to my goals as a triple jumper. Having a developed upper body definitely held me back and my athletics coach was constantly telling me that I needed to lose some of that mass because it was inhibiting my ability to jump, but for a while I basically disregarded his advice and kept doing what I was doing because it made me feel so good about myself. I did know that I was self-defeating to an extent, but the desire to build muscle and achieve a muscular physique was just as powerful as my desire to succeed as a triple jumper. When it comes to your body, things can get really complex, especially when you're a kid and still developing mentally and finding your sense of self, and I think a lot of it was tied to my self-esteem as well as my underlying preference to be a bigger guy.

By the third year of uni, I was training harder than ever. I'd moved into a student house for my second year, which meant two-hour round trips every day to get to training, which was far from ideal, and this, coupled with a sense of homesickness, meant that I moved back home again. I had started competing for a club by this point, would regularly represent the county and, the following year, I would be competing internationally for England. For the latter stages of university, I considered myself a full-time athlete as I was putting in at least a full-time job's worth of hours. But of course, as soon as uni ended I needed an actual job, one that paid a salary. Athletics is an amazing sport, and it taught me so much about training and my body, but in a financial sense it's about as lucrative as backgammon. It really is all or nothing. In Britain, unless you're one of the best in the world at your event, or very close to that category, you don't get paid a penny. I trained with other athletes who had won world championship medals and still didn't earn a salary. My athletics club paid for my transport and accommodation at events, and I got some free kit along the way, but I didn't earn anything from the sport. The sad truth is that across the country there are thousands of incredibly talented athletes who are working a full-time job alongside three or four hours of training a day, and the vast majority of them don't make it. Had I been at the equivalent level in, say, football I'd have been earning thousands of pounds a week, but, unfortunately, dwindling interest in the sport of athletics means that this situation is only going to get worse.

As soon as I graduated I got a job at a local gym as a fitness instructor, which really gave me an insight into how bad parts of the fitness industry can be. I absolutely hated it. I'd somewhat naively assumed I would spend most of my time training gym members, and thought it might even complement my own training, but in reality the 8–10-hour shifts, which comprised mainly of cleaning, where you were constantly on your feet just exhausted me and had a really negative impact on my performance, both in training and in the run-up to my athletics season. I had always put athletics first and I just couldn't do that at the gym. Don't get me wrong, I tried to make it work and I did everything I could to minimise the impact my job had on my training. I remember regularly delivering spin classes without even getting on a bike or sneaking into an empty studio to lie down when I should have been walking the floor. It sounds bad, but I didn't care – my focus was on becoming an Olympic triple jumper and I wasn't going to let anything stop me. By the time the athletics season came around, I actually decided to go part time so I had more time to train and could travel to competitions and recover better. Even so, I still felt the job was having a negative impact on my performance, and as I was living with my mum and youngest brother at this point (my parents had separated) my expenditure was pretty much non-existent, I decided to quit the gym job entirely. Although it was far from ideal to rely on my mum for food and accommodation given I was a twenty-two-year-old man, my desperation to make it as an athlete was so strong that I did it anyway.

I would say that I'm an ultra-optimistic guy, but there was definitely an element of delusion going on. Throughout my athletics career I set myself unrealistic targets, but I could never see that they were unrealistic. I always believed that the next jump would be massive and that the breakthrough was just around the corner. I would be hugely disappointed in myself when I didn't reach those goals, and that could sometimes make me feel pretty depressed. My overriding memories of my athletics career, particularly towards the end, was underperforming and always feeling that I could have done more. In 2010, when I was jumping for England, it felt like the momentum was building, but even though I often thought I was so close to nailing a career-defining jump, something invariably went wrong. That is the nature of triple jumping – there is a fine line between a huge jump and a complete disaster of a performance, but I definitely felt like I wasn't fulfilling my potential and that made a dent in my mental health over time.

I'd always been able to eat loads of food. My siblings and I share a freakish metabolism and I have vivid memories of getting home from school and literally emptying the kitchen cupboards, eating anything I could get my hands on. Sweet stuff was my preference and, looking back, my tolerance for sugary foods was immense. During my childhood I'd been constantly playing football, then as a teenager I built a lot of muscle mass and trained consistently, so by the time I hit my twenties, my body had essentially become a metabolic machine. But when the tension between what I was trying to achieve in athletics and the upper body mass that I'd developed really hit me, it triggered a bit of a crisis in my eating which would get progressively worse over the next couple of years. I'd basically got to a point where most things in my life had aligned to enable me to excel as an athlete, but my upper body and the unnecessary amount of muscle mass I was carrying was holding me back. Don't get me wrong, I wasn't huge. I was significantly smaller than I am now, but compared to the other triple jumpers I would compete against, I was like a giant, so much so in fact that officials at competitions would frequently mistake me for a discus or javelin thrower. Eventually, I decided that it was time to throw everything into the ring and really start to address the way that my muscle mass was detrimentally impacting my performance. I didn't want to look back and wonder what would have happened if I had lost a bit of weight – I didn't want to have any of those regrets. So it was clear I needed to lose weight and I thought I knew exactly how to do that.

The way athletics training works is that you spend the winter months building a foundation and work capacity, and then you gradually taper the training volume down in the run-up to the season, at which point you feel amazing. Well, that's the theory anyway. As jumpers and sprinters, we would build this foundation with horrible stuff like dragging tyres, or running up and down the dunes at Camber Sands – basically disgusting sessions which I dreaded and would inevitably end with at least one of the group violently throwing up. During this time I would eat a preposterous number of calories to aid recovery and help retain the unnecessary muscle mass I was so desperate to cling to. But then the summer competition season would come around, when I needed to be as light as possible in order to jump as far as I could. Competitions were always on a weekend, so I came up with a strategy whereby I would essentially starve myself Monday to Friday, lose a few kilograms, then come Saturday (and frequently Sunday too), immediately following my competition, I would give myself a window in which to eat. And when I say eat, I mean binge uncontrollably. All week long I would think about what I was going to eat after the competition, and it got to the point where I was more excited about the food I was going to eat afterwards than the competition itself. In the days leading up to an event, I would feel terrible and I remember literally having dreams about doughnuts because the cravings and hunger got so bad. So the minute the competition was over, particularly if I'd underperformed, I would go completely nuts. I'm talking competitive-eating style.

What started as one box of doughnuts on Saturday afternoon soon morphed into a non-stop binge lasting the whole of Saturday and Sunday. I would go to bed late on Saturday night to extend the period in which I could eat; looking back now, I would easily put away 10,000 calories a day over those weekends. Sometimes I wasn't even hungry when I was eating. Sometimes I felt so full, I could hardly move and would lie on my bed feeling like I was going to vomit. I remember thinking it was weird at the time, but I felt powerless to stop it. I had unwittingly fallen into a classic binge eating pattern, something which is common for athletes competing in sports which require a low body weight, but not something which a lot of people seem to talk about. I would lose 3–4kg during the week, then I'd put it all back on and sometimes more over the weekend. Of course, that meant that the cycle was absolutely futile. The reality is that it's almost impossible to lose that amount of fat or gain that amount of muscle in such a short period of time. When your weight fluctuates by such huge margins in a matter of days, those fluctuations are almost entirely down to changes in water weight. So, from Monday to Friday, all I was doing was losing kilos of water weight and emptying my body of valuable muscle glycogen stores, and then gorging myself on Krispy Kremes and pizza (or whatever else I could get my hands on) and gaining it all back in 48 hours. I would do that for the whole summer.

It definitely became a psychological thing that went way beyond just fancying a doughnut. My eating became tied to my emotional state. If I performed below my expectations at a competition, I'd be really pissed off with myself, so I'd immediately head to the nearest Tesco's or McDonalds drive-through. A lot of the time I didn't even really enjoy the food, it just became routine and I guess a desperate attempt to try and make myself feel better. There's a total lack of support for young people in a lot of sports, many of which encourage – if not actively then implicitly – some kind of starvation or significant restriction of diet, and I certainly fell into this trap. I know from the thousands of clients I've worked with that this kind of cycle can be all too easy to fall into, no matter what your lifestyle. If you do a crash diet once and it works, but you don't make any commitment to a more permanent change, you might be tempted to do it again, perhaps for a wedding or a holiday. Before you know it, you could be saving your calories all week for a blowout with your friends every weekend, then feeling absolutely terrible about yourself on Sunday evening, driving you to start the starvation cycle all over again. Or perhaps you spend the first six months of the year losing weight, then the next six months gaining it back, only to arrive back at square one. Many of us have a tendency to yo-yo and so many of us are overconfident about our ability to stick to plans which are entirely unsustainable.

For me personally, it was the all-or-nothing pressure of getting to a world-class level in athletics that crippled me mentally. I knew I only had a couple of years before I needed to start being an actual adult and thinking about life stuff like pensions and mortgages, so every week that went by where I didn't jump as far as I wanted to, or make the progress I needed to, the pressure just mounted. Looking back now, I definitely used 'crappy' food as a tool to combat this stress, but of course it only contributed to my feelings of failure.

As I mentioned, in 2010 it felt like things were on a bit of a roll, but in 2011 and 2012, everything went downhill.

Even though I was relatively talented, it just wasn't enough. To be a world-class athlete, particularly in the shorter, more explosive events, you've got to be a one in a million (possibly one in 10 million) genetic freak. I'm talking the kind of kid who wins the 100m at sports day by an absolute mile. And then does it again at district sports day, and then again at the county championships. I was good, but that's a different level. In hindsight, I was never going to be good enough to get to the Olympics, but the blindly optimistic side of me never really accepted that and instead I just pushed my body and mental state even further. In 2012, I ramped up my training yet another gear. My coach would send my training plan over to me and I'd spend hours methodically scrutinising every element of it and make so many changes that by the time I was finished it was unrecognisable from what I'd initially been sent. I absolutely loved the process of mapping out how my training was going to look for the next few months and seeing the linear improvements I planned to make, and that winter I remember training like an absolute lunatic, doing everything I could to get faster, stronger and more technically adept. As well as recording every minuscule detail of my training performance (and ensuring that I made numerical progress at every possible stage), I can also remember really focusing in on being lighter. By this point, I was acutely aware that achieving and maintaining a lower body weight was key if I wanted to be jumping the sorts of distances that I had planned. At this time, my weight hovered around 85kg and I was already very lean, but with the London 2012 Olympics coming up, I thought it was time to throw the kitchen sink at it.

Over time, I managed to completely change my perspective until I reached a point where the more muscular, bulky physique I'd had for the last few years no longer appealed to me. I remember starting to notice myself looking slimmer in photos, and whereas previously this would have made me feel insecure, I actually felt satisfied and happy in the knowledge that this new, skinnier physique was going to propel me to triple jumping success. I basically stopped all forms of bodybuilding overnight, and any weightlifting that wasn't specifically for triple jumping was removed from my programme. I very quickly lost a lot of body mass and became extremely lean. I dropped from 85kg to 79kg, which considering I didn't have much fat to lose was a drastic change, but for a triple jumper I was still bigger than the other guys. I continued to be locked in the starving and bingeing cycle, but it had developed to the point where I would drag out the period of starving myself for 10 days or two weeks. No matter what though, I would always, always eat like an absolute nutcase immediately after a competition. Both ends of the spectrum, the restraint and the release, got more extreme, and my longer periods of abstaining meant that my binges would become even more out of control. Knowing what I know now, I was in no condition to be training the way I was during those weeks of extreme calorie restriction. I would have been massively depleted in terms of muscle glycogen and overall energy – but back then I thought it was the only way I was going to succeed.

I did loosely understand that I needed energy to compete, so sometimes I'd starve myself Monday to Friday, and then the night before the competition I'd give myself a slightly bigger meal, generally in the form of a bowl of pasta, which compared to what I'd have been eating during the starving weeks was a good number of calories. The risk of this 'cheat' or 're-feed' system is that, in introducing a small amount of something you have been so desperately craving for so long, you end up experiencing a complete lack of self-control, and I remember this happening to me on a few occasions. Before one competition in particular, while staying at a friends' house in Nottingham, I had my standard pre-competition bowl of pasta, but ended up getting out of bed a couple of hours later to grab a snack, the whole time telling myself that it was fine and would help fuel my performance the following day. Before I knew it, I'd eaten a 1kg bar of chocolate in about three minutes, which probably eclipsed the total number of calories I'd eaten over the entire five days leading up to this point. It was as though when I started eating, I couldn't stop myself. Like literally couldn't stop myself. I'd know it was something I shouldn't be doing and that I'd be massively pissed off with myself afterwards, but the feeling of satisfaction I'd get from eating that particular thing was just too overwhelming to stop. Then within thirty seconds of finishing I'd be devastated and spend the night freaking out that I'd ruined the competition I'd trained so hard for.

In reality, it probably didn't actually make any difference and in comparison to the damage I was doing to my body week in, week out, it was a drop in the ocean. But for me at the time, it felt like a complete disaster. Those weeks would often be incredibly depressing and as well as being terrible to be around, I would end up going to bed early most nights rather than sitting around feeling hungry. I know I'm not the only one to have gone through that loss of control, and over the years I've spoken to other athletes, particularly bodybuilders, who have experienced similar things. A friend of mine told me that he once, while prepping for a bodybuilding show, woke up during the night and ate three whole boxes of cereal, before spending the rest of the night crying, knowing he had ruined weeks of dieting. It's like a force of nature when that level of craving hits you.

As weird as it feels writing this stuff down, I don't feel overly emotional or sad looking back at the food issues I've gone through. Perhaps because I haven't entirely taken on board how bad it got at certain points, but maybe also because I was always doing it *for* something, which made it feel somewhat legitimate, and the reality is that a huge number of people in sport, particularly in disciplines which involve any kind of limit or restriction on body weight, have to struggle with a version of my experience. Look at the boxer Ricky Hatton. He competed at a really low body weight, something that clearly didn't come naturally to him, and because he had to lose so much mass to achieve his fighting weight, he literally had two wardrobes. Ricky Hatton on the day of a fight versus Ricky Hatton a few months after a fight were literally unrecognisable. Living this cycle of starving and bingeing for years is really common, especially if you're psychologically conditioned, like I am, to overeat calorie-dense food on occasion. Having to restrict yourself for your sport, or even because you want to look a certain way, means that you are going to live half on and half off the wagon, with your weight yo-yoing, sometimes to extremes. That is why I would never compete in anything that required me to be a certain body weight again. I've spoken to people in sport who are literally nearly killing themselves, because they are starving so severely that their body begins to shut down and their hormones stop doing what they are meant to, all in the pursuit of something which, when it eventually arrives, is never as gratifying as they thought it would be. The irony is that, through social media, we often view images of athletes' bodies and assume that they must be healthy. Sportspeople can have totally aspirational physiques, but when you look at the flip side of how they have to live to get their body to look or perform a certain way, it is the opposite of aspirational.

There are also a lot of people living in this cycle who just don't talk about or even identify that their pattern represents unhealthy eating. I'm far more educated now, so I like to think that if I was ever in the same position again, I would behave in a much healthier way, but there would still be an element of restriction, and the truth is that there is no way I could stop myself from eating high-calorie, 'crappy' food for a sustained period of time. It's just not in me, and I know that personally any kind of strict limitation ultimately leads to the inevitable binge. So many of us are made this way, and it's why I believe so many diets fail in their ultimate goals. If you can see yourself in this kind of cycle and mentality, I just want to say, I've been there, and there is a way out – so keep reading.

It's definitely a taboo to talk about these kinds of things, especially the bingeing side, which culturally I think we wrongly associate more with a lack of discipline, when it is really a compulsion and an illness for many people. We just don't really share these types of experience; I think there is a level of shame and embarrassment around it, particularly with younger people. I'm pretty open as a person and I'm confident enough with myself that I don't care too much what people think about me, so it's easier for me to share what I went through. I'm also fortunate enough to be in a position to influence these kinds of conversations, and I definitely believe the stigma needs to be broken down. Just because people don't talk about it, doesn't mean it isn't hugely prevalent or that it isn't ruling and ruining people's lives. It just happens behind closed doors. Over the last two years, hospital admissions for eating disorders rose by over a third in the UK, but the true figure living with an eating problem is estimated to be way higher than that. In reality, hundreds of thousands of people across this country, and many, many more around the world, are suffering, and the truth is that, when it comes to disordered eating, it is chronically underdiagnosed and undertreated.

CHAPTER TWO

TRYING TO LOSE WEIGHT IS STUPID

If my own experiences with weight loss and weight gain, coupled with those of the thousands of clients I've worked with over the years, have taught me anything, it is to disregard most of what the fitness and diet industries tell you. And if I were to compile a list of common misconceptions which have come about as a result of this misinformation, right at the top of that list would be the whole concept of weight loss. If I had a pound for every person who has told me that they want to lose x amount of weight, I'd have a shit ton of money.

To be clear here: they don't want to lose *weight*. *You* don't want to lose *weight*. Unless you're competing in a sport that requires you to do so, no one wants to lose *weight*. What you actually want to lose is *body fat*. Almost every client I've ever worked with has at some point or another told me that they wanted to lose weight, when in reality it was body fat they were looking to shed. There's a big difference.

In case I've lost you at this point, let me explain what I'm on about. It is a question of body composition, not what the scales tell you. Your body weight is made up of an abundance of different organs and tissues. Body fat is one of those tissues, but so is muscle. And so is water. And so is your skeleton. And your heart, your brain, your lungs and every other organ for that matter. If you were to chop your arm off you'd lose a significant amount of *weight*, but unless you're an absolute psycho, this obviously isn't going to get you closer to your body goals. If you were to spend an entire day out in the sun and drink absolutely no liquid the whole time, you'd also lose a significant amount of *weight*, but again, this isn't something you should be striving for. Don't get me wrong, weight loss is often beneficial and a really useful indicator of fat loss, but it can also be incredibly misleading and a terrible gauge of progress during a diet.

I've worked with clients in the past who have changed their body shape completely, lost a huge amount of fat, drastically improved their health and fitness but lost almost no weight at all. In fact, I worked with one client (I'll refer to her as Anna Conda from here on in, but that wasn't her name) who actually gained weight despite losing a large amount of fat and looking a million times better. The reason for Anna's weight gain was that alongside her drop in body fat, she gained a significant amount of muscle mass. See, Anna had never lifted a weight in her entire life and so after six months of resistance training, her quads, hamstrings, glutes and pretty much every other muscle in her body had experienced hypertrophy (growth), while her stomach and waist had shrunk due to the drop in fat. And Anna's transformation isn't unique or unusual. The act of building muscle mass (which we'll talk about in Chapter 5) actually increases your metabolism, which in turn makes it significantly easier to lose body fat. A recent US study showed that dropping a few pounds of body fat and building a few pounds of muscle mass leads to an increase in metabolic rate of approximately 120 calories per day. And once you add in the calories burnt doing the exercise itself, the impact on your overall metabolic rate is huge. Basically, by doing resistance training alongside a period of fat loss, you'll end up looking strong and healthy, rather than weak and frail, which is something you typically find with someone who has just finished a crash diet coupled with no resistance training.

And while we're on the topic of weight loss being a ridiculous concept, BMI (body mass index) is also a joke. In case you're unaware of how BMI is calculated, it's literally your weight divided by your height squared. So the only parameters considered are your weight and height. That's it. As a result of this, my BMI is currently hovering around the 'overweight/obese' zone, whereas someone who is carrying a dangerous amount of visceral fat (fat which accumulates around the internal organs and isn't always externally apparent) but who has never trained in their life and has extremely low bone density could slot nicely into the 'healthy' zone. Great. Now, it has to be said that BMI isn't generally intended for athletes and can still be a blunt tool to help indicate whether an individual needs to lose fat, but it just goes to show how misleading BMI and your body weight as a whole can be. A far more relevant gauge is an individual's level of body fat (your body fat percentage), but this is extremely difficult to measure accurately, and your local GP doesn't have access to the necessary equipment to do so. So that is why BMI is still used.

In case you're still not convinced and are currently standing on your scales, methodically tracking your body weight while burning my book in a sacramental show of defiance, let me further stress just how deceptive your body weight can be. First things first, unless you are weighing yourself at exactly the same time, in exactly the same clothes, on exactly the same spot of floor each day, you are wasting your time. Let's break it down. Timing is massively important when you're weighing yourself. Say you wake up, step on the scales first thing in the morning and see that you're 80kg.

The following day you forget to weigh yourself in the morning, but you arrive at the gym after work and notice they have a set of scales. You've eaten well today and have kept yourself nice and hydrated, so you jump on the scales enthusiastically, only to be informed, much to your disgust, that you now weigh 83kg! You've gained 3kg in a day? Shit. But don't panic, you're not a fat wizard; it's pretty much impossible to gain 3kg of fat in a day. In fact, gaining 3kg of fat in a month would be an impressive effort. You have to overeat by approximately 3,500 calories in order to gain a pound of fat (around half a kilo), so an increase in body fat of 3kg would require an excess of 21,000 calories to be consumed. I don't care how much you think you like food, good luck with that.

So, if that's the case, how did you gain 3kg in a day? The answer is probably a combination of a few things. Firstly, you weighed yourself in the evening rather than the morning. This means that the food you've eaten over the course of the day is still mostly sat in your digestive tract, which will obviously add to your body weight. Additionally, the water you've drunk over the course of the day is incredibly heavy. A few glasses of water weighs around a kilo, and although you wee it out over time, it can hang around in your system for a few hours. On top of this, you're wearing clothes and trainers, easily adding another kilo or so to your total weight. Finally, the scales you're using are different to the ones you've been using at home. Believe it or not, the set of scales you bought from Asda for £9.99 might not be the most accurate device in the world.

And we're not done yet. Even assuming you're weighing yourself at the same time on the same scales each day, your meal and toilet timings can also have a dramatic effect on your weight. If on Monday you were to eat your final meal at 6pm and then wake up the following morning and rid yourself of that meal through the medium of your toilet, your weight would reflect this. If on Tuesday, however, you eat your final meal at 10pm and don't manage to go to the toilet before your weigh-in the following morning, that meal is still sat in your digestive system and as a result your weight will most likely be significantly higher. And *even* if you've got the meal and toilet timings nailed down, your levels of hydration can massively impact your weight on a day-to-day basis. Your body is made up of around 60 per cent water. Honestly, look it up. So, if you weigh 100kg, around 60kg of your body weight is water. Weird, right?! Anyway, this means that fluctuations in this level as a result of dehydration (not drinking enough water) or overhydration (drinking way too much water) can lead to discrepancies in body weight. Basically, you could spend a day eating junk food and doing no exercise whatsoever, but if you were to simultaneously stop drinking water (dehydrate yourself), it's completely possible that the following morning you'll have lost weight. And, once again, just in case you're in any doubt, this is not a good thing! Losing *weight* in itself is not necessarily a good thing. The fact that so many of us have spent years obsessing over the scales is one of the biggest failings of the government, medical, and health and fitness industries.

One thing that really blows my mind is when clients come to me and say something along the lines of, 'I want to lose two stone.' I'm always curious as to where this number has come from. Like, why two stone? Why not 2.5 stone? Or 1.75 stone? The answer is generally something to do with getting back to their weight when they were twenty-one, before they started their stressful job or had their first child and everything fell apart. Or simply because two stone is a nice round number. The bottom line is that this weight loss goal is completely abstract and ridiculous. Since when did your precise body weight matter when it comes to your appearance? When you see someone on the street or in a magazine who has a body that you aspire to, do you think, 'Ooooo, he must be 14.2 stone?' Or 'WOW! She's a solid 63kg!' No, you definitely don't. The point is, your body weight doesn't mean much. You could have two individuals with identical body *weight*, but one looks like an absolute Greek god or goddess while the other looks like they've just spent the last two years chained to an all-you-can-eat buffet. As a society, we tend to judge a person's physique based on their body shape, the amount of muscle mass they have, the amount of body fat they carry, where they hold their body fat, or a combination of all these factors. I'm not saying this is a good thing (it's what's on the inside that counts, and all that), but what is certain is that, outside of the sporting arena, no one has ever judged a person's physique based on their body weight.

And the same applies to your health. You could be classed as 'overweight' but be perfectly healthy, whereas someone else who is deemed to be a healthy body weight is actually anything but. The number on the scales when analysed in isolation is basically irrelevant. Using body weight as the barometer for the success of your diet, or the gauge with which to judge your health, is stupid and we need to stop doing it.

I used to look at the scales while I was starving myself and think, this is amazing, my weight is plummeting, I'm going to jump so much further! And yes, as a triple jumper, you do ideally need to shed unnecessary body weight to optimise performance. But if I were carrying two kilos more muscle and two less of fat, I would perform significantly better. The downside of fat loss is that it takes time and patience and happens at a slower rate than just a blanket loss of body weight. For long-term, sustainable changes to your body composition to take place, you have to make them over a longer period of time and do so in an incremental and, ultimately, boring fashion. That's another reason why many people in the fitness industry don't talk about the real, healthy and sustainable ways to lose fat – because generally, they suck! As I mentioned before, it doesn't help that tracking reductions in body fat is almost impossible outside of a lab, because unlike weight you can't see it on the scales. And before you tell me about the awesome new set of scales you just got for your birthday which track your body fat, I'm afraid they don't work. Or at least they don't work as a tool with which to measure your body fat accurately. You see, these scales operate by sending an electrical current through your body which has the ability to distinguish between lean mass (muscle) and fat mass. The problem is that this current will take the shortest route possible, which in the case of these scales means up one leg and straight down the other. So if you carry most of your fat on your upper body, you'll get a totally inaccurate measurement telling you you're way leaner than you actually are.

At this point, I know what you're thinking, why are you telling me to track my fat loss when there isn't an accurate way of doing so? I haven't got a science lab, mate. Don't panic, that's the beauty of fat loss: when you lose fat people will notice. You'll notice. Your clothes will get looser. Your waist will get smaller. Your skin will appear tighter and you'll look more 'toned'. Granted, you'll almost certainly float less when you go swimming but that's something you'll just have to learn to live with. Buy some armbands. Stick to the shallow end. Get really good at holding your breath. The possibilities are endless. The point is that losing fat is almost immediately noticeable both in terms of your appearance and the way you feel. But, in case you're an absolute nerd and you want a more tangible way to measure fat loss at home, like an actual objective measurement, that is also possible. I know I just spent ages telling you how terrible scales are (awkward), but you *can* actually track fat loss on the scales. As long as you know what you're doing and track other variables at the same time, your body weight can be a useful indicator of fat loss. For example, if you slightly reduce the amount of food you're eating, keep your water intake relatively high (and consistent from day to day), start resistance training a few times a week and your weight begins to drop slowly from week to week, congratulations! You're losing body fat! WOO!

So now we've got more of a handle on the theory, how does it work in practice? How do you actually go about losing body *fat*? Believe it or not, it's actually ridiculously simple. You put yourself in a caloric deficit. That's it. Game over. Stop reading. Throw the book out of the window immediately because we're done. Well, not quite. As simple as the process is, its execution can be extremely difficult. Particularly if you don't fully understand it. So, I'm going to make you understand it. You're welcome. A caloric deficit basically means that you eat less calories than you burn. So, if you're burning 2,000 calories a day, you need to eat less than 2,000 calories a day to start burning fat. Now you're probably wondering how to figure out how many calories you burn in a day. You may have just googled it. Don't. You'll find an abundance of websites that claim they can calculate how many calories you burn in a day (your metabolic rate). They can't. Unless you go to a science lab (again), no one can, and anyone who tells you otherwise is a liar. Or Gandalf. They're probably just a liar, though.

In reality, the best way to calculate your metabolic rate is simply by a process of elimination. Let me explain how this process works.

Day 1: Weigh yourself first thing in the morning (keeping all of the weigh-in variables we discussed earlier consistent). If you're an adult women you may likely eat, for example, 1,800 calories over the course of the day.[1]

---

[1] According to the NHS, an ideal daily intake of calories varies depending on age, metabolism and levels of physical activity, among other things. Generally, the recommended daily calorie intake is 2,000 calories a day for women and 2,500 for men.

Day 2: Repeat day 1.

Day 3: Weigh yourself first thing in the morning (keeping all of the weigh-in variables we discussed earlier consistent). At this point, there are three potential options:

1) If your body weight is now LOWER than day 1: repeat days 1, 2 and 3 but eat 2,000 calories

2) If your body weight is now HIGHER than day 1: repeat days 1, 2 and 3 but eat 1,600 calories

3) If your body weight is now THE SAME (within 100g) of day 1: congratulations, you've found your metabolic rate (it's 1,800 calories)

If you're a number 1 or 2 (your weight either increased or decreased), continue repeating this cycle, increasing or decreasing your calories by 200 a day, until you get to a point where your body weight stays the same over a period of a few days. At this point, the number of calories you've been eating per day is your metabolic rate and you now know how many calories you need to eat to maintain your current body weight. So, you simply drop this number of calories by 200-ish per day and you will begin to lose body fat. BOOM!

The problem is that as humans, it's not that simple. I know this from experience. Yes, sitting in a caloric deficit (consuming fewer calories than you burn) will result in fat loss. That's science; it's inevitable. However, *saying* it is significantly easier than actually *doing* it. Particularly when you love food as much as I do. How you go about achieving that caloric deficit has a huge impact on your long-term success. Essentially, if you go for the drastic, 'drop my calories by as much and as quickly as possible' approach, you'll lose loads of weight (notice I said *weight*, not fat) in the short term, but a lot of that weight loss will come from muscle and water.

In the body, every gram of glycogen (stored carbohydrate) is loaded with water, so when you drastically restrict your calories, you tend to also drastically restrict your carbohydrate intake, which results in your body breaking down its glycogen stores and you weeing out that water weight. Even if you are able to sustain this type of crash diet for a few weeks or even a couple of months, you'll inevitably revert back to your old eating habits at some point and end up ballooning back up to where you were before and probably beyond. The trajectory of crash dieting is completely predictable – it starts with an initial rapid weight loss, followed by a weight plateau, and then progressive regain. Weight regain is the typical long-term response to dieting for the majority of dieters. While you'll find stats on the internet saying that 90–95 per cent of dieters gain the weight back within a year or two (a lot of these stats are based on a very small study done in the 1950s of only 100 obese patients, but you'll still see them repeated in pretty much every diet book), we still don't have definitive percentages on success and failure. It's also difficult to compare like for like: a thirty-year-old woman who is just on the edge of being overweight versus a clinically treated morbidly obese man would obviously have different challenges when it came to maintaining weight loss. But what we do know from research overviews of over twenty-five long-term weight loss studies is that this pattern of rapid weight loss, plateau and then weight regain is the rule not the exception.

So, if crash diets don't work, how about 'elimination diets', the newest buzzword from our ever-evolving (to screw you out of more money) diet industry? If you go for the 'tomorrow I become a monk and will never look at anything containing sugar for the rest of my life' approach, you are setting yourself up to fail just as much as the crashers. Everyone can resist the things they like for some time, but realistically, you're not going to keep it up forever. You'll be out for dinner with your friends, or you'll have a shitty day at work, or your housemate will leave some doughnuts unattended in the kitchen, and it's game over. And when I say game over I mean you'll eat everything in the house because you've eaten one doughnut and ruined it, so what's the point any more? You can start afresh tomorrow so you might as well just 'get it out of your system'. Right? Whatever you tell yourself, the truth is that your diet sucked and that's why you fell off the wagon. To be honest, you shouldn't have been on a wagon in the first place. You don't need a diet to lose fat. You need to understand how fat loss works and then change your lifestyle sufficiently to allow this process to take place without losing muscle.

I skirted over it there, but the faster you reduce your calorie intake, the more muscle mass you will lose. And muscle mass plays a key role in enabling you to burn lots of calories, and for some people is a desirable look. We know it takes a deficit of approximately 3,500 calories to lose a pound of fat, so obviously you can't achieve that in a day or two. However, if you reduced your calorie intake by 500 a day, say from 2,500 to 2,000, that would equate to a drop of 3,500 calories over the course of a week, and the loss of one pound of fat. If you find that kind of underwhelming, weigh out a pound of butter and imagine cutting it off your stomach. It's a huge amount of fat to lose. Yet often you'll see guidelines from the diet industry suggesting you should be losing two pounds or more a week. And just in case it's unclear, losing two pounds of fat in a week would require a drop of approximately 7,000 calories. That's 1,000 fewer calories every day – a level so low that there is no doubt your muscle mass, glycogen stores and energy levels would take a big hit, which, as mentioned above, ends up being counter-productive in the goal of long-term fat loss. I know it's frustrating, but we just need to slow things down.

The other major issue when it comes to losing fat is that your metabolism isn't something that is static. In fact, it is incredibly adaptive, which is one of the main reasons behind the extremely annoying yet incredibly common plateau phase in weight loss. Numerous studies have shown that a reduction in calorie intake over a period of time (a diet) leads to a reduction in the number of calories an individual burns. Say you reduce your calorie intake by 1,000 calories overnight. What will happen is that firstly, you will lose water weight from glycogen and muscle alongside a bit of fat too, and that might happen very quickly, especially if you have a lot of mass to lose. But the side effect is that your body will freak out and assume it's being starved. This process, brought about by that drastic drop in calories, repeated continually over time, will result in a temporary change in your metabolic rate. So instead of continuing to burn calories at the same rate as you were at the beginning of the diet, your body will do everything in its power to protect your vital organs and prevent you from starving to death. It sounds dramatic, but if you were to lose a pound a week for a few years, you'd die. Obviously. There would be nothing left of you. That is why your metabolism adapts to prevent this, and that is also why diets stop working over time. Those 1,500 calories of green tea, yoghurt and salmon that were working so well at the start of your diet are no longer enough to lose fat. Your body has got used to that caloric intake and adapted accordingly, clinging to those 1,500 calories as if your life depends on them, because from its perspective, it does.

You see, the body craves an equilibrium. A state in which everything is ticking over nicely and nothing is too taxing for it. What you've inadvertently done is killed your own metabolism, and the irony is that you're now in a position where not only is it almost impossible to lose more fat, but when you return to your 'normal diet' – the one you were eating before you started losing weight – you'll gain weight and the never-ending yo-yo dieting cycle begins.

Something else we hear little about – as well as presenting misinformation, I would argue that the diet industry suppresses certain research because it doesn't suit their intention of extracting money out of you – is how calorie deprivation absolutely massacres your body's hunger hormones. A drastic reduction in calories reduces the levels of leptin, known as the satiety (fullness) hormone, which helps regulate your long-term food intake. A caloric deficit (and indeed fat loss) will lead to you feeling progressively less full when you finish your meal, and obviously the more extreme your calorie crash, the more extreme the dip in the hormone. At the same time, it boosts the levels of ghrelin, aka the hunger hormone, which stimulates your appetite, increases food intake and promotes fat storage. The result of a crash diet is that your body is desperate to get the hormones back on track, back to that equilibrium, so it will pump out ghrelin while restricting leptin until you are as hungry at the end of a meal as you were when you started. One study showed a 24 per cent increase in ghrelin in a crash dieter's blood plasma over the space of six months. No matter how incredible your willpower, that is literally your body willing you to ruin your diet.

Instead, if your meals consist mainly of whole foods, enough protein to retain (or perhaps even build) muscle mass and provide a sense of fullness, and include 'good' fats such as those found in avocado, for example, you will find that the ghrelin levels decrease and as a result that clawing, absolutely gutting sense of permanent hunger will fade. And if you add in fibre, exercise regularly and get a good night's sleep, you'll increase your leptin levels too, ensuring that your body doesn't foil your best-laid plans. For both of these hormones, the very worst thing you can do is decimate your calorie intake in a short period of time. Doing so is like jumping off a moving train because you want to get to your station quicker. It's not going to happen, mate.

I know it sucks that you can't do this quickly. But trying to do it all in the space of a couple of weeks or even months, will back you into a corner and doom you to long-term failure. No one wants to tell you this and I would love to say I could give you instant results. But it's only by dropping your calories slowly and eating a diet high in protein and fibre, while ideally implementing some form of resistance training, that you can reduce your body fat in a long-term, sustainable way. I'm not saying that you'll *never* be hungry on 300, 400 or 500 fewer calories a day, but it will be to a much lesser extent and you'll find it far more manageable than if you were to slash 1,000 calories off your daily intake.

What I generally find is it's the growing, insatiable hunger that builds from these hormones on top of cravings for things that you are missing that kill most diets. Just like me, most people cannot bear to totally cut out calorie-dense (and delicious) foods. The best way to avoid hunger and cravings is to change the way you eat, focusing on foods that fill you up by taking up space in your stomach, but costing you the fewest number of calories. Say you aim to eat 1,500 calories a day. Yes, you could do that at McDonald's and still potentially lose fat. But you will find yourself hungry for more food all day. Fifteen hundred calories of McDonald's equates to a Big Mac, large fries and a milkshake. I know that if I eat only that, I feel like I want to eat more (and more and more). If, on the other hand, you made up those 1,500 calories from chicken breast, rice and vegetables, you will feel like your stomach is going to explode, and eating more of anything will be the last thing on your mind. If you don't believe me, try it. Put 1,500 calories of McDonalds next to 1,500 calories of chicken breast, rice and vegetables and see what impact each has on you.

Now, I know what you're thinking: McDonald's is nicer than chicken, rice and vegetables, and I couldn't agree more. I'm not going to lie to you and tell you that some kind of magical conversion is going to take place whereby you turn into Gwyneth Paltrow and prefer chicken, rice and veg to a Big Mac. I mean it might, but it's unlikely. I'm also not saying you should never eat McDonald's. In fact, if you enjoy eating McDonald's, I think you should definitely eat it. *Just don't eat it all the time.* And drop your calories a little over the next few days to level things out. But, as a general rule, the best tactic is to go for massive fibrous, protein-dense foods. Try making a 700-calorie salad with some lean meat thrown in. The sheer amount of food will be huge and after eating it you'll feel full because the protein will stop your stomach from emptying quickly and the fibre will stop your leptin levels from plummeting. Contrast this with 700 calories of chocolate brownie, which won't even touch the sides, and you'll see what I mean. Dropping your calories to lose fat isn't enough – you need to understand which calorie sources are going to make your life easier and eat them as often as possible.

Aside from the leptin factor, fibre is often hugely underestimated in terms of its impact on the success of a diet. Fibre is extremely bulky, which means that it fills your stomach and helps to prevent overeating. In addition, when you eat it, the gut bacteria in the intestines ferment compounds which trigger other appetite-suppressant hormones. That's why eating good sources of fibre, such as brown and wild rice, wholewheat pasta, bulgur wheat and seeded wholemeal bread is so useful. You'll also find fibre in fruit, vegetables, beans and lentils, so chuck all of that into your salad, too. Then there are things like mushrooms, which have a variety of fibres including mucoprotein and resistant starch, which are really hard for your body to break down and cause your stomach to expand while slowing the process of it emptying.

As for protein, there's been a lot of controversy about how much we actually need, especially for muscle growth.

Bodybuilders and strength athletes tend to go over the top with their protein consumption, but there's no doubt that it plays a crucial role in fat loss. A lot of the controversy has focused on animal products as a convenient source of protein, but there are plenty of non-meat proteins like beans, lentils, nuts, soy products and wholegrains out there too. While the exact optimal amount of protein for muscle growth is unknown, as a general rule, and within reason, the more you can fit into your diet the better. Good sources of protein are essential for tissue repair, as they tend to be full of amino acids, which are the building blocks of muscle. Their presence in the body is fundamental in this process. Studies also show that the thermogenic effect of eating high-protein foods (the production of heat as a result of eating) means your body has to work harder to digest it and therefore *just by eating protein*, you burn significantly more calories than if you eat carbohydrates or fat. It has also been proven that a protein-rich diet will lead to a higher percentage of fat loss to muscle loss, so in short, keeping your protein topped up will mean you retain more muscle while shedding a higher percentage of fat, even if your calories remain the same.

Essentially, eating a diet that is high in both protein and fibre is like using a cheat code on the Xbox. Do it. (The diet, not the cheat code. Nobody likes a cheat.)

CHAPTER THREE

HOW TO EAT DOUGHNUTS AND NOT GET FAT

Many of the clients that come to me have been dieting on and off for years. Some of them have been eating a really low-calorie diet for most of their adult lives. The irony is that despite eating so few calories, a lot of them are overweight (they're carrying too much body fat). Generally, their story goes something like this: they've lost weight at some point in the past, but after a particular crash diet or just a period of long-term calorie restriction, their metabolism crashed and now they are completely stuck. They also have a relatively low level of muscle mass and this, combined with their damaged metabolism, means that they are finding it almost impossible to shed fat. They often feel their only option is to drop their calories even lower, but realistically, unless they want to spend their life eating the diet of a three-year-old child, that just isn't going to be possible. Although at this point all seems lost, there is a solution. In fact I'm amazed that more people aren't aware of this particular strategy, because it's a literal lifesaver: the answer is a *reverse diet*. This is a tool that could potentially help millions of people stuck at a dead end due to a broken metabolism as a result of dieting, as well as those who have struggled with an inherently slow metabolism their whole life.

The premise is simple, the execution less so, just because it takes a really long time and is pretty painstaking. But it does have the power to help you create a great 'forever' body. In essence, the idea is that you train your body to handle more food – you literally force your metabolism to stop being a dick and start burning more calories.

What takes a bit of wrapping your head around if you've been raised on faulty diet myths, is that, to an extent, the more you eat, the faster your metabolism will work. Since I was a teenager, or even before that, I've always eaten a lot of food because I have always been active and relatively muscular, and that has driven a fast metabolism. Getting kids into sport and fitness at a young age really pays off in the war against obesity, because you help them build a healthy body composition (high muscle to fat ratio), which in turn fuels a faster metabolism. Going into adulthood, I've been able to train my body to continue to burn calories at a really high level, but if you took the average person off the street and gave them my diet for six months, they would almost certainly gain a huge amount of fat, because that's not what their body is used to or capable of processing efficiently. Crucially, this metabolic adaptation also works the other way: the less you eat, the slower your metabolism will become. As we discussed in the previous chapter, this is one of the biggest reasons that most diets fail.

Imagine a guy (let's call him Harry Balzak) decides to go on a crazy crash diet in an attempt to lose loads of weight before a holiday to Spain with friends in eight weeks. Harry wants to look great on the beach and awesome in pictures, so he decides that to lose weight, he needs to seriously cut his calories. He's only got eight weeks, so he doesn't want to hang around. Harry typically eats 2,200 calories a day, but he slashes that number to 1,500 calories a day. Week one, he loses loads of weight on the scales and he feels great, even though we know that the majority of what he's lost is water and muscle, which is actually detrimental to long-term fat loss. Week two he might lose a little less, and he's probably starting to struggle a bit mentally, but he's still feeling happy with the results. Somewhere over the next few weeks, however, things go downhill fast. Harry's still only eating those 1,500 calories a day, but his weight on the scales has stopped going down. Why? How can 1,500 calories lead to weight loss one week and not the next? The answer is actually very simple. Initially, anyone who starves themselves will lose body weight. But a month or so in, in an act of self-preservation, Harry's body has adapted to the reduced number of calories, his metabolism has slowed down accordingly, and those 1,500 calories that worked so well at first are no longer sufficient to lose weight. Without wanting to sound too scientific here, Harry is basically fucked. If he wants to lose more weight, he's going to have to drop his calories even further, perhaps as far as 1,200 calories a day, and for an adult male to be eating 1,200 calories a day, despite what some so-called nutritional experts will have you believe, is absolutely ridiculous.

See, before he embarked on his ill-fated crash diet, Harry was cruising along, comfortably maintaining his body weight while eating 2,200 calories a day. But he's now eating just 1,500 calories a day and still maintaining his body weight. He's effectively trained his body to be less efficient at burning calories, and what's more, in the act of losing weight so quickly, he's also lost a significant amount of muscle mass. This post-crash diet fallout that Harry is experiencing is a position that millions of people around the world have found themselves in at one point or another. You decide you want to lose weight (actually fat) or continue losing weight (actually fat), but you can't seem to drop your calories low enough for the number on the scales to start shifting. Or the number of calories you'd need to drop to in order to start losing fat just seems stupidly low. To all intents and purposes, you're stuck. Enter the reverse diet.

A reverse diet is exactly what it sounds like. It's the opposite to a standard diet. Instead of gradually *reducing* the number of calories you eat in order to lose weight, you gradually *increase* the number of calories you're eating – over time, and painstakingly slowly. The painstaking element is crucial here, because if you increase the calories too quickly, you'll just get fat. The trick is to find that sweet spot between eating the same number of calories and nothing changing, and eating too many calories and your body storing it as fat. Now don't get me wrong, during a reverse diet you'll almost certainly gain a small amount of fat – that's inevitable as you're putting yourself in a caloric surplus. But by increasing your calories slowly and consistently over a sustained period of time, you give your body the stimulus it needs to get better at burning calories, without giving it so many calories that it just stores them all as fat. What's also amazing about this process is that, unlike a traditional diet, because you're in a very slight caloric surplus, your body is capable of building muscle mass at the same time. This means that, if executed properly, and run alongside some form of resistance training, six months or so down the line you'll emerge from your reverse diet with a significantly faster metabolism and a much healthier (and better looking) body. You'll potentially have a little bit more fat, but the increase in muscle mass will often give the illusion of having lost fat and, crucially, you'll have turned your body into a calorie burning machine. At this point, you'll be able to lose fat relatively easily, eat a lot more food without gaining fat, and the best part is, you'll understand how it all works. You'll be in control of your body and you'll have the power and knowledge to change it if you choose to.

A reverse diet is by no means an easy fix, however. It's not a short-term process and this is probably why it isn't as widely used as it should be. You've got to commit to a long period of time where you'll have to track your calories each day (actually pretty easy to do these days) and you won't be losing weight (fat) in the process. It's not something you can implement before your holiday to drop a few pounds, and you'll have to demonstrate a level of self-discipline in order for it to work (though I'd argue it needs significantly less self-discipline than eating a miserably low number of calories while yo-yo dieting for most of your life). It could take anywhere from a few months to a year to get there, but the end result is something so amazing that I promise you it's worth it. When it comes to long-term, sustainable change, there is no shortcut.

So how do you physically implement a reverse diet? How many calories do you need to eat and for how long? Let me explain.

The first thing you must do before starting a reverse diet is to establish your basic metabolic rate (the number of calories you need to eat for your body weight to stay the same). We discussed this process in Chapter 2, so that shouldn't be a problem. You also need to weigh yourself three times a week (ideally space these weigh-ins out, e.g. Monday, Wednesday and Saturday), keeping all of those weigh-in variables consistent. Remember, hydration, the time of day, your toilet activity and meal timings can have a dramatic effect on your weight, so make everything as similar as possible. Once you've completed your three weekly weigh-ins, you're going to take an average of those three figures and that will be your weight for the week. Even when keeping your weigh-ins consistent, your body weight can still fluctuate, so by taking an average we allow for any unusual activity on the scales. If you're unsure of how to take an average, literally add the numbers from your three weigh-ins together and divide the total by three. So if your numbers were 80kg, 81kg and 80.5kg, your total would be 241.5kg, and that divided by three is 80.5kg. Therefore, your average body weight for the week would be 80.5kg. Now it's time to begin the reverse diet.

Week 1: Add 100 calories to your daily calorie intake.

Week 2: If your weight drops, stays the same, or goes up by 100g or less, add another 100 calories per day. If your weight increases by more than 100g, continue with the same number of calories.

Week 3: Repeat week 2.

Week 4: Repeat week 3.

And that's it! You simply continue this process until it stops working or you feel like you've increased your metabolism sufficiently.

Sounds simple, right? It is. Well, in theory anyway. Obviously implementing it in reality and fitting it around your life may not be the easiest thing in the world, but as I've already mentioned, it's 100 per cent worth it. It also has to be said that by the time you're finished with your third or fourth cycle of the ridiculous crash diet you read in a magazine once, you could have just done a reverse diet and be sitting in a far better, astronomically more smug position.

I've talked a lot about calories, and they are obviously fundamental to the success of your reverse diet, but where are those calories going to come from? We know that keeping your protein and fibre high will make things significantly easier on the diet front, but what about the other macronutrients – fats and carbohydrates? There are so many schools of thought out there when it comes to the consumption of these. There are people who follow a keto diet and would rather die than let a single gram of carbs pass their lips. They'll tell you with complete confidence that carbohydrates are the devil and will make you fat overnight. Conversely, there are people who follow a low-fat diet because they're convinced it's impossible to eat fat and lose weight. The truth is, rather disappointingly, that in the long term, the ratio of carbs to fats in your diet makes no difference whatsoever. A study in *The New England Journal of Medicine* concluded that any reduced-calorie diet will result in weight loss, and that the percentage breakdown of macronutrients within the diet doesn't mean a thing. Basically, as long as your protein is high (for reasons already discussed) and your calories are where they need to be, the percentage of carbs and fats you choose to eat is just that: your choice. Some people find that eating lots of carbs makes them sluggish, whereas others need to get a good source of carbs in before going to the gym in order to feel good, but when it comes to losing and gaining fat, calories (and to a lesser extent protein intake) are king.

In case you're unsure of what I'm saying here, or you're still convinced that eating carbs before bed will make you fat, let me lay it out for you once more. Assume Person A and Person B both need 2,000 calories to maintain their body weight. Person A eats 2,000 calories a day with 250g of carbs, 50g of fat and the rest from protein. Person B eats 2,000 calories a day with 125g of carbs, 110g of fat and the rest from protein. Because these two individuals are eating the same number of calories and a very similar amount of protein, the impact on their body composition will be the same, despite the difference in the amount of fat and carbs in their diet. That's it. It's that simple. Everything you've read about carbs making you fat is a lie. The only area where carbohydrate intake can impact body weight is on an acute (short-term) basis and if you've learnt anything so far, I hope I've made it clear that's ultimately irrelevant. If you lower your carbs drastically, you will lose weight quickly, because as we discussed previously, every gram of stored carbohydrate in the body is loaded with water and so a reduction in carbs leads to a reduction in water weight. But this weight loss is nothing to do with body fat and, over time, the level of water weight within the body will return to normal anyway.

Another thing I should throw into the ring at this point is micronutrients. I know I've said that calories are king, and that aside from protein, how you fill those calories is irrelevant, and that's true as far as your body composition goes. However, in terms of health, micronutrients are extremely important. Micronutrients are the vitamins and minerals that we need in various quantities to maintain a good level of health. They are consumed in far smaller quantities than macronutrients, but are key when it comes to the way our bodies function on a daily basis. Micronutrients such as vitamin C, zinc and magnesium play a crucial role in boosting our immune system and reducing our risk of illness and so shouldn't be neglected. Eating a diet rich in fruit, vegetables, wholegrains and lean protein sources (e.g. chicken breast) will pretty much cover you on this front; supplementation (see Chapter 6) can also be adopted for convenience.

So, to summarise, you can eat doughnuts and McDonald's and still lose fat, as long as you keep your overall calorie intake below your daily calorie requirement. However, while junk food can be an adequate source of macronutrients, it's never going to be an adequate source of micronutrients, and so the implications of your diet on your long-term health as well as your body composition is something that shouldn't be overlooked.

I touched briefly on the whole 'carbs before bed making you fat' thing, and this is another huge misconception within the fitness and diet industries. Countless studies have proved that meal timings and frequency are ultimately irrelevant when it comes to body composition. One recent Canadian study concluded that 'increasing meal frequency does not promote greater body weight loss'. In short, when you eat your meals, or how many meals you eat, makes no difference. If you eat 2,000 calories a day, it doesn't matter whether you eat those across three or six meals. Similarly, it doesn't matter whether you eat your final meal at 6pm or 11.27pm.

And the same goes for the plethora of diets out there that claim to have magical fat loss properties. They don't. Following a keto diet won't directly lead to fat loss. Intermittent fasting also won't directly lead to fat loss. Going vegan? You guessed it, this also won't directly lead to fat loss. The only thing that directly leads to fat loss is a reduction in your calorie intake (eating less) or an increase in your calorie expenditure (exercising more). That's it. Now, that's not to say that following a particular diet won't help you achieve that reduction in your calorie intake. I myself have tried intermittent fasting in the past, a diet that includes limiting your eating to a particular window within a day, and found it very useful. I'm never hungry first thing in the morning and so by skipping breakfast and instead eating my first meal at lunchtime (a form of intermittent fasting), I found achieving a calorie deficit far easier and was able to lose fat. But, and this is crucial to understand, it wasn't intermittent fasting that made me lose fat. It was *eating fewer calories*. If you go vegan and lose fat it's not being vegan that made you lose fat, it's the fact that you started eating fewer calories. Being vegan may have helped facilitate this reduction in calories and therefore fat, but it was the reduction in calories alone which led to the fat loss.

And while I'm destroying myths like a massive, shredded Jonathan Creek, I might as well eradicate a few more.

'Eating healthy food makes you lose weight.' It doesn't. Apples are 'healthy' but if I eat 500 apples a day I'm going to gain weight (and eventually die). Conversely, I could eat nothing but Dominos pizza, but if I keep my overall calorie intake below my daily requirements, I'd still lose fat. If you need more proof, just ask Mark Haub. As a professor of Human Nutrition at Kansas State University, he spent ten weeks eating nothing but Twinkies, chocolate bars, powdered doughnuts, Doritos, sugary cereals and Oreos. Crucially, however, he kept his overall calorie intake below his daily metabolic rate. The outcome? He lost 12kg, lowered his 'bad' cholesterol (LDL) and increased his 'good' cholesterol (HDL). He also reduced his level of triglycerides (a form of fat) by 39 per cent. Admittedly, he was taking additional vitamin and mineral supplements, but this experiment alone demonstrates that it's ridiculous to label one food 'good' and another 'bad'. There are no good and bad foods, especially without context. A cheeseburger can be good if it's incorporated into a healthy, balanced diet, and as I've just explained, apples can be bad if you eat too many of them. If someone commits a murder while wearing a green T-shirt, it doesn't make green T-shirts bad.

'Sugar is bad.' It's not. I've eaten a diet high in sugar for my entire life and I'm healthy. Sugar won't make you bigger or stronger or healthier, but it also won't stop you from being any of those things. Eating too much of it might, but eating too much of anything also might. That isn't a sugar problem, it's a moderation problem. 'But sugar causes diabetes.' It doesn't. In fact, Diabetes UK (the British Diabetes Association) even states on its website that 'no amount of sugar in your diet – or anything in your lifestyle – has caused or can cause you to get Type 1 diabetes', and that 'we know sugar doesn't directly cause Type 2 diabetes'. When it comes to high-sugar diets, although you'll spend a lot of time (and money) at the dentist, it's the associated increase in calories that causes you to gain fat, not the sugar itself.

'What about eggs? Eating eggs is bad for your cholesterol, right?' It's not. A number of studies have shown that the dietary cholesterol found in eggs is not actually absorbed very well by the body and so doesn't affect our levels of cholesterol.

I'd like to think you can see where I'm going with this, and I could go on all day, but I won't. The point is that the fitness and diet industries are absolutely rife with misconceptions, so learning how your body works and responds to food and exercise is key to overcoming the absolute quagmire of shite out there.

CHAPTER FOUR

STOP USING YOUR INJURY AS AN EXCUSE

Right, I'm bored of writing about your diet, so let's get back to the most important topic here: me. (That was a joke.) A lot of you probably don't care about my background but I've got a word count to hit so you're going to hear about it. Unlucky. We left my athletics career on a bit of a high: although my diet and approach to food in general was pretty messed up, my performances were improving and I had aspirations to compete at the London Olympics in 2012. Unfortunately, things were about to take a turn for the worse, and the lessons I learnt during that time are significant for anyone who has ever been injured, whether from exercise or from an accident outside of sport. I've lost count of the number of people I've met who've used a previous or existing injury as an excuse for not being active, or as the reason for them being overweight. The truth is, it's not an excuse, and inactivity is almost always a result of laziness or a lack of desire to change (unless you have a pre-existing mental or physical condition). This is something we'll come back to later in the book.

In 2012, I was training like a lunatic. At the start of the year I was ranked third in the UK, but only the top two would qualify for the Olympics, assuming they met the required standard. Although in reality I was miles off this standard, being the optimistic guy I am, I genuinely believed I had a chance. I threw everything I had left into my training and diet, hitting the track or the gym six days a week, sometimes twice a day, and spending every waking hour plotting how I was going to improve my jump. I had continued to get leaner and lighter as a result of the extended periods of calorie restriction, and things were starting to look really good with my distances in training and my numbers in the gym. I started to feel a sense of fulfilment, that all of this sacrifice was beginning to pay off.

But my lower back decided it had other plans. As a triple jumper you're almost constantly injured, and success in the sport often comes down to who can manage those injuries best, so when my back started aching during sessions, I didn't pay much attention to it. When an elite level athlete performs a triple jump, during the hop phase in particular, they load their body with up to *twenty-two times* their own body weight – so an 80kg athlete temporarily weighs in at around *1.7 tonnes*. Triple jumpers have been called the 'ultimate Olympians' as their shin and thigh bones often become thicker, developing into what has been described as a super-skeleton in order to withstand the huge amount of pressure they're put under. Basically, it's like jumping off a three-storey building, and as you're landing on one leg at a time, it's very unilateral, which means that as well as developing an imbalance in your physique, your ankles, knees, hips and back get absolutely pummeled.

Most of the time, my many minor injuries would just go away by themselves; I learnt that an element of 'just getting on with it', as outdated as that sounds, actually works really well (within reason, obviously). You see, most people's natural reaction to an injury is to stop and do nothing, which in a lot of cases is the worst course of action you can take, as I will show you later in this chapter. But after a few years of not being able to stand still for more than five minutes because of pain in my lower back, the problem that I'd been 'managing' wasn't getting any better. In fact, it was getting worse. Initially, I'd feel it if I landed a jump awkwardly, then it would carry on after training, but eventually it got to the point where, after finishing a jump session, I'd have to lie on the sofa for three or four hours because I couldn't stand up without excruciating pain. I remember after one monster jump session in particular, the next day I couldn't get out of bed. I mean, if we're being pedantic here, I could've rolled out and fallen on to the floor, but you know what I mean.

It turned out that I had prolapsed a disc in my lumbar spine. You can google it if you want a bit more info, but basically my back was fucked. I had a couple of scans and my physio said I'd probably had it for a while, but with the intensive training it had got progressively worse and was now at the point where jumping or even running was no longer possible. The actual prognosis was to stop doing any activity that involved any impact on my back, i.e. pretty much everything. Great.

It was soul-destroying. I'd gone through months of grueling preparation, endless disgusting training sessions, as well as all those weeks of starving myself to try and lose weight. And now, to top it all off, I could barely move; I had a few weeks where I was literally stuck to the sofa, as the pain was so intense. Mentally it was an incredibly hard time and I would say I was genuinely depressed. As I couldn't extend my spine, there was no chance that I would be running or jumping any time soon. I actually had to develop a modified, semi-bent-over walk just to be able to get around. And even when the pain started to subside and I was able to walk normally, the chances of me being able to compete again were non-existent. With the triple jump, there can be no hesitation. You can't hold yourself back. If you want to jump a long way, you need to be 100 per cent committed to the take-off, and with the state of my back, this was never going to happen. I felt as though every ounce of air had been knocked out of me. This had been my life for nearly ten years and I couldn't come to terms with the fact that I might never do it again.

After a month of bumming around on my sofa doing very little, I started to accept the situation and began to look for a more positive side. I'm a relentlessly optimistic person, and this helped me pull myself out of the hole I was in. I'd also just spent four months starving myself and obliterating my body on the track and in the gym, so there was definitely a sense of relief that I could just kick back, eat 'crappy' food and do whatever I wanted (as long as it involved lying down). Sairs and I (her name is Sarah but her family are weird and love giving each other shortened names which I've now inadvertently adopted) were also engaged by this time and we'd had to put off the wedding because I hadn't wanted it to interfere with my competition and training schedule that summer – triple jumping had been the main priority in my life to that point, so everything else had come second. But when I realised I wouldn't be able to compete, we decided to get married that year, which was obviously amazing and gave me something positive to focus on. It took time, but I did start to see the light at the end of what had been a really long and pretty shitty tunnel.

My athletics career taught me a lot about how the body heals and how to adapt and work around injuries, and this, coupled with my degree in Sports Therapy, meant that I developed a solid understanding of most injuries and how to cope with them. I also learnt just how far you can push your body. I was doing stupid amounts of training, and after the sessions I'd often be an absolute wreck, lying on the floor completely ruined. But your body does recover; in fact your body possesses an unbelievable capacity to adapt and overcome nearly anything – it's literally designed to do it. If you don't believe me, ask any woman who's ever given birth. Or a manual labourer who spends ten hours a day working in a way that would ruin the average person after twenty minutes. At the start of every winter, I'd have training sessions that would end with me throwing up and then falling asleep at 8pm because I was so tired, but within a few weeks, these same sessions were a breeze. This is adaptation, the process your body undertakes which enables you to get better at stuff and do more. This same process can be applied to injuries and their rehabilitation, but the fundamental aspect in all of it is the stimulus that you give your body to adapt to. Too little and the healing process will take forever, but too much and the injury will simply get worse. While we are often told that an injury may never heal completely, and that the affected area might never be the same again, in most cases, a full recovery is 100 per cent possible and in my experience, the rehab process can actually be used as an opportunity to make the injured site stronger than ever.

You will no doubt have been told – possibly by medical professionals – that rest is the most important thing when it comes to injury. Put your feet up. Do nothing. Avoid putting any pressure on it. Now, I am in no way suggesting that anyone with acute pain should be going to the gym – you have to listen to your body and really get to know what works and what doesn't when you have an injury. But absolute rest for all but the most extreme injuries – think a broken leg – will invariably result in a slower and less complete recovery. For the majority of injuries, particularly those most common among people who exercise regularly (soft tissue injuries relating to muscles, tendons and ligaments), this advice is actually at odds with the way the body heals.

If we take a super common injury, such as an ankle sprain, the structures involved are the ligaments and sometimes tendons of the ankle. Through some kind of trauma (usually rolling your ankle on an uneven surface), a tear has occurred in one or more of the ligaments. (A sprain is just another word for a tear, by the way.) Now, many structures in the body, particularly tendons and ligaments, have a poor blood supply and this means that when you are injured, after the initial swelling has subsided, the affected area is going to take a long time to heal. A good blood supply is crucial for the healing process to take place, and the better the blood supply to the injured area, the faster the healing process will be. But sitting down with your feet up definitely won't stimulate a good blood flow to the area – quite the opposite in fact – and this is where the stimulus and adaptation process comes in. Numerous studies have shown that gentle exercise helps speed up healing and can also be helpful for improving balance and stability and reducing the risk of reinjury.

So the classic advice to 'just rest' a minor injury is actually the opposite of what you should do, and even if rest does eventually lead to recovery, the chances are that when you return to being active, the injury will reoccur. This is down to two things. Firstly, you probably haven't assessed the real cause of the injury, and there is always a chance that it may have been caused by an underlying biomechanical issue, particularly if it came about over time and not as a result of a sudden impact or accident. So, if, for example, you decide to start the 'couch to 5k' but after a few weeks of running most days of the week you begin to get pain in your knee, the chances are that this is caused by an underlying flaw or imbalance in the way you run. It may be that you pronate (roll in and flatten) your feet when you run, and over time this can lead to stress injuries of the feet, ankles, knees or hips, particularly when running on hard surfaces. You might have been doing it your entire life and had absolutely no idea, but if you don't rectify this underlying issue, as soon as you return to exercise, the injury will almost certainly return. These kinds of stress injuries are most common in people who perform repetitive movements for long periods of time, such as walking, running or cycling and so, before anything else, try to identify the biomechanical issue that caused the injury.

Secondly, if you do nothing with that injured knee other than sit around for a few weeks with your feet up, you're effectively telling your body that you don't need your knee to be strong, mobile or resilient; you simply need it to be able to rest on the coffee table while you watch Netflix every evening. The end result will be a weak, stiff knee which is highly susceptible to reinjury. If, however, you slowly begin to mobilise your knee, performing weight-bearing, proprioceptive (balancing) exercises which progressively increase in difficulty, not only will the increased blood supply speed up the healing process, but you'll end up with a knee which you're far less likely to injure in the future.

As I mentioned earlier, this is something of a balancing act, and just as doing nothing is bad for recovery, doing too much is even worse. Fundamental to being able to manage this process is your ability to gauge pain. Here, there is also a lot of confusion and mixed expectations around pain, particularly in relation to fitness. There is this idea that pain is bad and something to be avoided at all costs. People automatically assume that pain is an indication of injury, and so they stop what they're doing at the first hint of discomfort. This is probably one of the main reasons why the active approach to injury rehab that I've just talked about is avoided by most people, because they're scared of pain. In reality, pain can be a great indicator of progress. Obviously, excruciating pain during rehab or exercise is not a good thing and should be avoided at all costs, but if during your mobilisation exercises on your injured knee, you get some low-level pain which loiters annoyingly but doesn't really get any worse, that's absolutely fine and actually shows that you're pushing your body to adapt. You're providing a stimulus and telling your body that you want your knee to heal so that you can use it to do stuff. When it comes to rehab and exercise as a whole, it's all about moderating your volume (how much you do) and learning what type of pain is acceptable, and what is dangerous and to be avoided. Being unable to make this differentiation is something which holds thousands of people back and prevents them from making the progress they so desperately crave.

Now, you may have got to this point in the chapter and be wondering what this has to do with your desire to lose a bit of body fat and improve your body composition. The answer is nothing. You've literally just wasted half an hour reading a few pages of utterly irrelevant information. This is awkward. Jokes. It has everything to do with your body goals and how you're going to get there. As I've said countless times, in order to lose fat and/or get the body of your dreams, you're going to need to do some kind of exercise, ideally in the form of resistance training. And over time, the chances are you'll incur some form of injury, which is the excuse that hundreds of people have given me in the past for them being overweight or not making any progress. The thing is, it's a rubbish excuse. Unless you're completely incapacitated, an injury can be managed and you can still make progress towards your goals in spite of it. It won't be easy and it might hurt at times, but that just makes the outcome even more rewarding.

So, what does this process actually look like? How do you go about creating a rehab plan for yourself? Let's take my back injury as an example. The NHS estimates that up to

80 per cent of people will experience back pain in their lifetime, so if you've been dealing with something similar, hopefully this story will help you reassess some of the myths you've been told or picked up unconsciously along the way. When I hurt my back, I knew from all of my experiences of injury that sitting for weeks or even months in a chair wasn't going to help me. Of course, I had to rest at the beginning, because I was in a lot of pain and there was a significant amount of inflammation around the injury, but I knew that as soon as I could, I would need to start moving and begin the process of stimulus and adaptation.

The back injury itself wasn't a one-off; it had been building up over a period of months, possibly even years and had been causing me chronic pain. At the time, I'd genuinely forgotten what it felt like to train without pain in my back, so I decided that it was worth investing everything in it to make it bulletproof. My goal was to make my lower back so strong and resilient that I would be able to do whatever I wanted – possibly even triple jump again – without pain. I essentially started training like a bodybuilder, but with the focus on maintaining perfect form for every exercise that I did. I kept the weight light and didn't allow my technique to break down at any point, particularly with exercises involving my back. I began to eat significantly more food, because that is an incredibly effective way to speed up the muscle-building process. As mentioned before, your body wants to do the absolute minimum to achieve equilibrium or homeostasis, so it doesn't want to build muscle. Why would it? The more muscle you have, the more work it's got to do to maintain it. In order to convince your body to build muscle, you have to firstly give it a significant stimulus (resistance training), and secondly the means with which to actually build the extra muscle tissue – this comes in the form of a calorie surplus (eating more calories than you burn).

Initially, I used resistance machines and focused predominately on training my upper body as this caused me the least discomfort and, due to the seated nature of the equipment, offered my back a degree of protection. As well as the desire to strengthen and rehabilitate my back, there was also the latent desire to build some serious muscle mass, as there had been throughout my teens and early twenties. After a couple of months of this style of training, the pain in my back was much less noticeable and I felt confident enough to ramp things up. I started by combining my hypertrophy training (training designed to build muscle) with incredibly light compound movements using a barbell. Whereas an isolation movement is one involving a single joint with a focus on a single muscle (e.g. a bicep curl), a compound movement involves more than one joint and therefore more than one muscle (e.g. a squat). Compound movements are more beneficial than isolation movements because they offer you more bang for your buck, but they are also more taxing and typically involve at least a degree of pressure on your back. Given my situation, this was obviously a risk, but I decided that by keeping the weight incredibly low, the risk would be minimal. I decided to focus, in particular, on the squat, bench press and deadlift.

With my squats, I began with no weight at all, just performing the movement with my own body weight. With the deadlifts, I would literally use the bar alone (your typical gym bar weighs 20kg). Bench press was less of an issue as it involves almost no loading on your lower back, so I was able to lift a little bit of weight there. After a few weeks of familiarising myself with these three movements, building a foundation of strength and mobility, and, crucially, becoming semi-confident that my spine wasn't going to explode, I began to take things up a notch. I would do five sets of five reps for each of the exercises, always keeping the weight at a level which gave me zero discomfort and allowed me to execute each rep with perfect technique. Now, I'm an impatient guy, so to say that this process sucked would be an understatement. It was painstaking and I definitely had to swallow my pride. There were so many occasions when I wanted to lift heavier and I felt like the other guys in the gym were laughing at me, but I knew I was doing the right thing, and after a few weeks of lifting next to nothing, my back continued to improve. It was working!

After celebrating the fact that I was an absolute genius, I started to increase the weight on a weekly basis. I would literally go up by the smallest increment possible, which in my gym was 5kg. After a month or so of back-pain-free progress, I realised that this linear model of progression wasn't going to work for much longer. What you'll find at most gyms is that they'll have plates which go 25kg, 20kg, 15kg, 10kg, 5kg and then 2.5kg. If you're lucky you might even find some 1.25kg plates but that's as low as they'll go. The problem with this is that if you want to increase the weight, you have to make a jump of at least 2.5kg (1.25kg on each side of the bar). This is fine at first, but after a while, unless you're a robot, you can't continue to progress at these increments. That's just not how humans work. And given my need to protect my back, this was even more of an issue for me, so I invested in some fractional plates. These are plates of lower weight than those you'll find in your gym. They're basically designed for absolute nerds like me who also like lifting weights. The set I bought went down as low as 0.2kg, which literally looked like a pair of CDs but allowed me to increase the weight I was lifting by smaller increments each week. As if I didn't already look weird enough lifting just the bar, I now would regularly turn up to the gym carrying a bag of tiny micro plates.

I know I joke about it, but I'm very aware that people going to the gym for the first time, or first few times, will feel pretty intimidated. It's not just becoming familiar with the machines or working out in public; often it's the other people that can make you feel uncomfortable and, particularly around the free weight areas, you end up having to work out around a lot of big guys. This was how I felt as a teenager venturing into the gym for the first few times, and then again when I began my rehab process and had to spend most of my time lifting the lightest weights I could get my hands on. I think the thing to remember is that generally other people don't give a shit about you. I don't mean that in a depressing way, I just mean they are generally focused on themselves, which means they're just not looking at you. And even if they are looking at you, the chances are they're not doing so in a negative way. These days, if I see someone who is clearly new to the gym, I think 'good for you', or more often than not I don't even notice them because I'm too busy training myself. When I see someone overweight running, or someone skinny trying to build muscle, I think what an absolute hero, because that person has probably been through a lot to get to this point and they're doing something they're probably not completely comfortable with in order to better themselves. If you can't applaud that then you're a bit of weirdo.

Often our perceptions of people looking at us are more to do with our own paranoia than reality. But if there are people who laugh at you or make negative comments, the best way to deal with it is to feel sorry for that person. After all, someone who is happy in their own life would never project that kind of negativity on to someone else. I think you have to have a level of empathy with people like that because they are clearly in such a terrible place in their own life that they have to think badly of you to make themselves feel better. Anyone who is overly critical or takes the piss is venting their own negative energy, betraying their own unhappiness and projecting their own insecurities. I'm happy with my life and where it's going, so I don't ever have the urge to be horrible to someone for trying to better themselves. I've got better things to do with my time.

What I will say is that unfortunately there are going to be hurdles on the way to achieving your body and fitness goals. It sucks that you might be made to feel embarrassed at the gym, but it's not always going to be emotionally comfortable or easy to get to where you want. If it *were*, you wouldn't be in this position in the first place. I would also mention that if you keep going to the same gym a couple of times a week, those feelings will go away. I promise. I can vividly remember my first trip to the gym as a sixteen-year-old with a couple of mates and the feeling of just complete awkwardness at not having any idea what to do or where to stand. I can remember bench pressing for the first time and hating it because it felt so unnatural to me, but those feelings are temporary, and you get over them. I guarantee that even if you absolutely hate your first experience of the gym and never want to go back, if you persevere and stick to a plan, before you know it, you'll gain confidence in yourself and stop worrying about what you look like to anyone else there. Or at least worry a lot less so that it doesn't stop you wanting to go.

As for my progress, I kept bringing my nerdy micro plates to the gym each week and slowly increasing the weight across all of my lifts. I resisted the urge to chuck loads of extra weight on the bar and was constantly mindful of my technique above all else. It wasn't immediately rewarding and was actually consistently frustrating, but over time my numbers began to creep up and after a year or so I had built a good amount of muscle mass from the hypertrophy training I'd been doing alongside my strength training. Without really realising it, I'd been following an unbelievably basic, but incredibly effective form of progressive overload, a principle that underpins any successful training programme. I'll go into more detail in the next chapter, but simply put, progressive overload involves making your training harder over time. In doing so, you provide your body with a stimulus to adapt to and in turn it gets bigger, stronger, fitter or all of the above. I did this by making ridiculously tiny jumps in weight each week across my lifts for the best part of a year.

This brings up the question of patience. How the hell did I keep going when it was so long-winded? There were a couple of factors that helped. In addition to rehabbing my back, I was also training other areas of my body, which meant that I could see more tangible results. If my back was supported, it was possible to train my arms and other areas of my body, and I had a lot of fun with that and could pretty quickly see a change in my physique. And to be fair, even though the rehab work was light and boring, it was still gratifying because I was making progress; I could literally feel my back healing.

For me, it was another massive lesson about the body. As with dieting, slow and steady wins the injury race. I didn't shock my body into anything, I always kept within my capabilities and just took things step by step without ever jumping ahead of myself. Increasing weights in small increments always felt safe and manageable, and because I started at such a low weight, it felt as though I could progressively overload forever. I never got to the point where I was struggling to lift the weight and therefore never put my back at any risk. Although we've established that injuries require a stimulus to adapt and that sometimes this stimulus can be uncomfortable, staying in the safety zone is essential; it's very much a balancing act and pushing too much too soon will simply send you straight back to square one.

Obviously there will be cases where someone genuinely can't achieve their body goals due to injury. But for the vast majority of people who have suffered injuries and as a result stopped exercising and gained weight, there is no real excuse. We've already touched on the fact that there are going to be barriers in the journey. The harsh truth is that it is up to you to decide whether you want it enough. If you say to me, 'I *can't* train or exercise three days a week because I don't have time,' that's a lie. What you're really telling me is that training and getting in better shape isn't enough of a priority in your life, that it's not important enough for you to find the time to do it. If I offered you £1,000,000 to go and sit on a chair for an hour, three times a week I guarantee you'd find the time to do it. Why? Because it'd be important enough to you that you'd find a way. Even if it meant waking up at 3am to fit it in, you'd be sat on that chair three times a week. So the next time you tell yourself that the reason you haven't been to the gym for a month is that you haven't had time, stop lying to yourself and admit the truth. You don't care enough about changing your body to actually do it. And that's fine by the way. You don't have to change anything if you don't want to. But if you're telling me that you do want to make a change then you better be ready to do something about it.

The truth is, if you don't care enough, you won't do it. You say you want to lose fat, but do you really? Is it just an idea that would be nice, but actually if you're being honest with yourself, you're not prepared to confront the barriers ahead? There are going to be so many hurdles to jump to get what you want, so before you invest money in a gym membership you won't use, think to yourself: do I really, really want to do this? If you do, you're going to have to go through awkwardness and discomfort, both mentally and physically, but the payback will be that you come out the other end with a body composition that you didn't think was possible. That decision is something that you need to take ownership of and responsibility for. Somewhere along the line, a company has marketed something to you, whether it's a diet or a fitness plan which will have made you believe that something or someone else is responsible for helping you reach your body goals. The reality is that it's you and you alone who will determine how your body looks and feels, so stop looking for excuses.

Woah. That was intense. Anyway, after a year of taking control of my injury, I was loving life. I was training five days a week, I wasn't getting injured, I was looking forward to going to the gym and I never dreaded sessions. I felt so much stronger than when I was a triple jumper. Back when I couldn't stand up for more than five minutes without my lower back aching and was in a constant state of injury and pain management. But now my back felt stronger than ever and that made me feel so incredibly liberated and gratified that I'd made that change myself. All the responsibility and the achievement was mine. I felt more comfortable in my own skin and was way happier within myself.

Despite this satisfaction with the position I now found myself in, I started to feel like I was lacking direction. I felt ready for a new challenge. Coincidentally, around this time, it dawned on me that the three lifts I'd been focusing on so heavily for the past twelve months – the squat, bench press and deadlift – were the three lifts which make up the sport of powerlifting. I started to look into the sport and actually went to watch a local competition and was immediately hooked. In hindsight, it's quite a weird thing to get hooked on: loads of people screaming at each other while straining under ridiculously heavy weights, but I thought it was awesome, and the camaraderie among the lifters definitely appealed to me. I had started to miss the competitive nature of athletics and craved something more exciting than just my routine gym sessions, so I decided there and then that I was going to become a powerlifter.

BOOM! First cliffhanger of the book! Bet you're literally scrambling to find the next page as we speak.

CHAPTER FIVE

HOW TO GET BIGGER, FITTER, FASTER AND STRONGER

After a year of painstakingly slow progress, I had finally reached a point where I no longer viewed my training as rehabilitation. I hadn't experienced any significant back pain for a long time and my focus had slowly shifted from trying to fix my back, to simply wanting to get as strong as I possibly could. I would say around this point that I definitely got addicted to the feeling of getting stronger. In many ways it was perfect for my mindset: it was completely objective, I could track my progress on my phone and see this diagonal line going upwards, which I always derived a huge amount of satisfaction from. Like a creepy amount. Imagine Norman Bates sat on a rocking chair in a dark room studying line graphs. That's what I'm talking about. I never actually did that, but I am quite weird. Anyway, after another few months of slightly more aggressive progression, I was the strongest I'd ever been, my back was the best it had ever been, and I was lifting more weight than I'd ever lifted. And the coolest thing about it was that it didn't even feel that heavy. I'd followed the purest, most linear form of progressive overload, and in case you're unaware, progressive overload is *everything*. If you only take one thing from this book when it comes to exercise, it should be how to use the principle of progressive overload.

We've already established that progressive overload is the process of making your training harder over time. And just in case I haven't stressed this enough, it's absolutely integral if you plan to make any kind of progress. In short, if you exercise for any period of time and aren't mindful of progressive overload, you're basically wasting your time. In my case, I achieved it by slowly increasing the weight I lifted each week, but there are loads of ways you can go about it. You can do more reps, have less recovery time, train harder, more frequently or for longer – the possibilities are endless. The key is to continually increase the training stimulus so that your body knows that it needs to adapt. So what does this actually look like in real life? Here are a few examples:

Example 1 (a twenty-year-old male who's just started going to the gym):

Week 1: Chest press machine for 3 sets of 8 reps with 20kg
Week 2: Chest press machine for 3 sets of 10 reps with 20kg
Week 3: Chest press machine for 3 sets of 12 reps with 20kg
Week 4: Chest press machine for 3 sets of 8 reps with 25kg
Week 5: Chest press machine for 3 sets of 10 reps with 25kg
Week 6: Chest press machine for 3 sets of 12 reps with 25kg

Example 2 (a forty-three-year-old female who's just started running):

Week 1: Run for 5 minutes three times a week
Week 2: Run for 5½ minutes three times a week
Week 3: Run for 6 minutes three times a week
Week 4: Run for 6½ minutes three times a week
Week 5: Run for 7 minutes three times a week
Week 6: Run for 7½ minutes three times a week

Example 3 (a thirty-two-year-old male who's just started strength training):

Week 1: Squat, bench and deadlift for 3 sets of 8 reps @ 70% of one rep max*

Week 2: Squat, bench and deadlift for 3 sets of 8 reps @ 72.5% of one rep max

Week 3: Squat, bench and deadlift for 3 sets of 7 reps @ 75% of one rep max

Week 4: Squat, bench and deadlift for 3 sets of 7 reps @ 77.5% of one rep max

Week 5: Squat, bench and deadlift for 4 sets of 6 reps @ 80% of one rep max

Week 6: Squat, bench and deadlift for 4 sets of 6 reps @ 82.5% of one rep max

* Your one-rep max is the most weight you can lift for a single repetition of a given exercise

Now these are all extremely basic models of progressive overload, and each example (particularly 1 and 3) would require more exercises to be added in order to make a complete training plan, but following any one of those examples would result in you getting better at that particular thing. If you don't believe me, try it. And then come back and apologise for being a distrustful little weasel. Sorry, that was harsh. I'm just really passionate about progressive overload.

So why does slowly increasing the difficulty of something make you better at it? To be honest, it's an incredibly basic process and simply involves capitalising on your body's constant need to adapt. If we look at the woman in Example 2, in week one she runs for five minutes three times a week. This is tough and her body is freaked out by this new, stressful stimulus. Fortunately, however, the relatively short nature of the five-minute runs is manageable, and by repeating them three times in that week, she's given her body a chance to adapt without pushing it so much that it begins to break down. Come week two, she runs for five and a half minutes, and although this increase of thirty seconds per run is enough to force her body to adapt once more, it's a small enough jump that she's still able to manage it without absolutely killing herself. Fast-forward to week six, and after repeating this process for four additional weeks, she's now running for seven and a half minutes three times a week and she feels great. Her body has evolved to suit the demands she's put on it. It's realised that it needs to get better at running and so that's exactly what it's done. Her lung capacity has increased, her heart is stronger and more efficient, her joints and muscles are more resilient, and her running technique has improved. And all of this has taken place in just six weeks. Nuts, right?!

Now, let's contrast this with another individual who decides to jump in at the deep end and go for a twenty-minute run right off the bat. They manage to drag themselves along for the duration of the run but are absolutely ruined for the next few days. Fortunately, they managed to avoid injury but due to the soreness (and memory of how much the run sucked) they decide not to run again for a couple of weeks. Although they've battered their body, some adaptation will have taken place, but because they waited another two weeks to run again, by this point the adaptations have faded and they're back to square one. They feel guilty for not having run for two weeks and so go for another monster twenty-minute run. This time, halfway in, their body can no longer cope with the stimulus (it hasn't had a chance to adapt to it) and this manifests itself in the form of a pulled hamstring. The individual is now unable to run for six weeks, they gain weight, and the never-ending cycle of failed attempts to get fit begins.

The key difference between these two cases is that the woman in the first example built her runs up gradually, whereas the individual in the second example did pretty much the opposite. This slow, incremental form of progressive overload is crucial for long-term, sustainable results. By keeping the progression slow and sub-maximal, you stress your body enough to force it to adapt, without stressing it so much that it can't cope and injury or regression occurs. You also 'keep something in the tank', which allows you to continue progressing for longer. I mean, I literally increased the weight I was lifting pretty much every week for an entire year! That type of linear progression is almost unheard of, but with a sensible, sub-maximal approach and an enormous amount of patience, I was able to increase the weight on the bar each week, while rehabbing and strengthening my back at the same time. The key is to make progress doing the least amount of work possible. If you can get stronger by going to the gym once a week, do it! Then further down the line you can add in a second session and so on.

At this point, it's also worth highlighting the importance of consistency in your training. We know that you need to make things harder over time to allow progressive overload to take place, but you also need to keep the exercises you're doing relatively similar in order for the stimulus to be sufficient enough for adaptation to take place. If one week you lift weights, the next week you go for a run and the following week you play snooker, your body won't have a consistent stimulus to adapt to and you won't make progress. That's not to say that you shouldn't try different things, just try to make them part of a bigger, more consistent and structured plan.

Anyway, back to my new sport of powerlifting. So, what exactly is it? As I mentioned before, the sport is made up of three lifts: the squat, the bench press and the deadlift. At a competition, you have three attempts for each lift and it's actually fairly similar to the jumps or throws in athletics, whereby everyone takes it in turns with a view to lifting more weight with each attempt. Then, once everyone has had their three attempts for each lift, your best squat, bench press and deadlift weights are added up and the person with the biggest total wins. Simple. But beyond that things get a bit convoluted. Unlike football where you have one governing body (FIFA), in powerlifting there's friggin' loads, and they all have their own unique rules and standards. The sport started back in the 1960s, but has never gained Olympic recognition, mainly because of the different factions and lack of unity. The International Powerlifting Federation (IPF) is the most recognised of all the different organisations, and it also mandates drug testing, which a lot of the other organisations don't. It was for this reason and the fact that the IPF attracts the best powerlifters in the world that I decided to join this federation. It was really important to me that any competition I was going to enter was based on real, drug-free strength, plus you have to ask why someone would choose to compete in a non-drug tested environment – it looks pretty sketchy, right?

I actually quite enjoy talking openly about drugs, because it's something that anyone who has an impressive physique, particularly on social media, is often confronted with. Bodybuilders, powerlifters, weightlifters, strongmen and women, whoever – if you have a good amount of muscle mass, and particularly if you're also pretty lean, it's presumed by many that you've taken steroids to get there. There is no doubt that drug use is incredibly prevalent in the fitness industry. If you are looking at professional, competitive bodybuilding for example – a discipline based entirely on aesthetics, and which is now frequented by the biggest, most ridiculously muscular humans on the planet, individuals who have almost become caricatures of themselves – it's fair to say that a lot of them are probably getting some 'assistance'. That's not to say that they wouldn't have had incredible physiques without taking drugs, because they definitely would – to get to the elite level in bodybuilding you need to possess one in a million genetics, but that extra 'supplementation' has enabled to them to exaggerate their already abnormal features and become these people whose mutant-like bodies have to be seen to be believed.

But a lack of education and understanding about the way these drugs work is one of the main issues facing the fitness industry today. The problem is that people, particularly young males, see anyone with a decent physique and assume that the only way to achieve a similar body is to take drugs. More often than not, they've only been training for a few months, haven't been eating enough food, and have no idea what they should be doing in the gym, but the modern-day society-wide issue of impatience and wanting to achieve amazing results without putting in the work leads them to use drugs as an excuse. 'That person only looks better than me because they're taking drugs.' 'I'd look that good if I started taking drugs.' The reality is that these body-builders would still be freaks without drugs, because they have inherited the most insane genetics for muscle growth and symmetry – the drugs are merely the icing on the cake; the element that gives them that extra 5 or 10 per cent they sadly need to compete in the modern era. They are already the anomaly, the 1 per cent, but because they've taken drugs, we've lost sight of the fact that 95 per cent of their body is down to their DNA, diet and training. Just in case you're still unclear here, you don't take steroids and wake up the next day massive. That's not how it works.

Anabolic steroids mimic the effects of testosterone, which is the primary male hormone that promotes muscle growth. If you're interested in how it actually works, you have to look at various elements. Firstly, testosterone increases neurotransmitters which encourage tissue growth; it also interacts with receptors in DNA which encourage protein production; and finally it increases levels of growth hormone, which does exactly what you imagine it would. So, are they legal? Well, in the UK the answer is yes and no. Steroids are a class C drug and are prescription only. The grey area is that it's not illegal to possess them for personal medical use, but it is illegal to sell them. By law, you're not allowed to post them, receive them by post or buy them online. Even giving them to your friends is considered supplying (54 per cent of people say they got their steroids from a mate). Breaking the law comes with a maximum fourteen-year prison sentence. And obviously, if you're caught using them in any professional sport, you'll be banned, potentially for life.

So how come so many people use them? We've all seen the documentaries of labs in Russia manufacturing drugs for their Olympic teams, and we all know the truth about Lance Armstrong – but that's just elite athletes, not your regular guy in the local gym, right? Sadly, no. These days, you can find steroids everywhere. The National IPED (Image and Performance Enhancing Drugs) info survey in 2018 revealed that a million men were using steroids in the UK, mostly to improve the way they look, with over 50 per cent saying they used them for cosmetic purposes. And it's not just twenty- or thirty-year olds – even kids as young as thirteen are getting their hands on them. Public Health Wales estimates that 350,000 male users aged sixteen to sixty-four visit needle exchanges across England, Wales and Scotland due to steroid use. I know a number of individuals who don't compete, aren't particularly big or muscular by current fitness industry standards, but who've taken drugs because of the pressure to look good on social media. I don't judge any adult who's made the decision to take steroids: if that's what you've decided to do and you're happy to take the risks, ultimately, it's your body. What I do question is the way they are taken so quickly, before people give their body the chance to reach its natural potential. There are people who've been training for three months who think, right, I've been doing this for a while now, I haven't seen much progress, I must need drugs to get bigger. This is absolutely ridiculous. Like literally mental. You need to train for years to get anywhere near your natural potential, and even then I still wouldn't advocate their use. The risks to your long-term health are huge – we're talking heart issues, an increased risk of prostate cancer, kidney and liver problems, mental health issues, not to mention the impact on your sleep and sex drive, and if that wasn't enough, taking steroids will literally shrink your balls and make you go bald. Not so tempting now, right?

Another issue with the use of drugs, particularly on social media, is that, in a lot of cases, individuals aren't open about their drug use. The result of this is that people cannot accept or conceive that you can have a body like mine without taking drugs. Granted, I have good genetics for muscle shape and symmetry, and I'm bigger and more muscular than the average guy, but I'm not a freak by any means. My physique is completely attainable for anyone with similarly decent genetics who is willing to train as effectively and for as long as I have. But even when I was competing as a powerlifter and going through semi-regular drug testing, people just wouldn't believe that I didn't take drugs. This misconception can be pretty frustrating at times, but ultimately people are entitled to their opinion and when you really analyse it, they're paying me an enormous compliment. What they're essentially saying is that my physique is so impressive that I couldn't possibly have achieved it without drugs. Thanks, guys!

What does bother me, however, is the thought of a sixteen-year-old kid following me and assuming that they need to take drugs to build a good physique. This isn't the case, and you can build an amazing physique, a body better than you ever thought possible, without taking anything. I'm living proof of this, and there are thousands of other examples out there too. But don't expect it to happen in a few months, or even a few years. It's taken me fifteen years and I'm still trying to improve. You've got to be prepared to play the long game, so stop looking for excuses and start making a plan.

So, I joined the IPF because it drug-tests competitors, but also because it attracts the best lifters, meaning that's where you'll find the highest standard of powerlifting. I did my research and found a competition that was happening in a few months, a couple of hours from where I lived, so I signed up and everything went from there. The powerlifting community is an incredibly supportive environment. You might imagine that all these massive men and women lifting hundreds of kilos are totally unapproachable, but I've always found the exact opposite. My first competition was still a huge eye-opener though. All I can say is that until you do it, you can't be prepared for it. I performed pretty well on the day and ended up hitting a couple of huge PBs (personal bests – the most weight you've ever lifted), but I also messed up quite a bit in the form of a few red lights. Basically, at a competition, as you lift, you are surrounded rather awkwardly by three judges, each sat on a chair. There are a number of intricate rules for each lift, and if any one of the judges deems you to have broken one of those rules, they'll give you a red light. If, however, they're satisfied that you've completed the lift within the rules, they'll give you a white light. You need to get a white light from two of the three judges in order for your lift to count. Most of the rules are understandable, but some of them are quite harsh and can result in a seemingly successful lift being disqualified on a technicality. For example, if you successfully complete a squat but put the bar back on the rack before the judge gives you the signal to do so, the lift doesn't count. Despite

115

this, I was instantly hooked. The feeling of grinding out a huge deadlift while the other lifters and an audience of spectators scream at you to get the lift is an unbelievable feeling and something I definitely miss today. If you enjoy lifting (or trying to lift) heavy weights in the gym and are looking for a sport to get involved in, I can't recommend it enough. To be honest, I would probably still be doing it today if it weren't for one thing: the amount of food I had to eat to get to the top of the game.

After all that starvation and pressure to lose weight that I experienced throughout my triple jumping career, you'd have thought I'd be keen to do the exact opposite. And when I first started powerlifting, I was. I drastically increased my calories and loved the freedom it gave me with my diet, and of course the resulting increases in strength. But after a year or so of competing, eating shitloads of food and loving life, my body weight had plateaued and was seemingly stuck around the 95kg mark. At this point I was faced with a choice: I could continue to hover around the same body weight and accept that although my strength progress would be slow, I could eat what I wanted and enjoy the process, or I could put everything I had into gaining weight and getting as strong as my body would physically let me. You probably know me well enough by now to know what choice I made. Obviously, I decided I was going to try and become the strongest human the world had ever seen, and I was going to do it quickly. And to get stronger quickly, you have to eat more. Like, a lot more.

If you look at strongmen and women, you'll notice that while they carry a huge amount of muscle mass and are typically absolute giants, they also carry a lot of body fat. You see, within reason, the greater the calorie surplus you create, the faster you will build muscle and strength. The problem with this approach is that you also gain a lot of body fat. There's basically an optimal level of extra calories that will lead to the most muscle gain possible, but beyond that point your body simply can't build muscle any quicker and so the rest of the surplus calories will just be stored as fat. It's like painting your house blue. The first couple of coats will make it blue, and then the third coat might make it a little bluer, but coats number four, five and six will make no difference. Your house can't get any more blue at this point and the extra paint is just making the walls thicker. Also, you're going to look like an absolute weirdo going into B&Q and buying that much blue paint. And who even paints their house blue? What would the neighbours think? Anyway, you get the point. The thing with strongmen and women is that they don't know exactly where that optimal level of blue paint is, and so they'll chuck another couple of coats on just to make sure it's as blue as possible. And they can afford to, because carrying some extra body fat is actually fairly useful in a sport where body weight can help generate momentum and create force. After all, there are no weight classes in the World's Strongest Man or the World's Strongest Women – the bigger you are, the more weight you're going to lift, so why wouldn't you get as big as possible?

The difference with powerlifting, however, is that it does have weight classes, and sitting around the 95kg mark, I'd automatically slotted into the 93–105kg category. One option I had was to drop down into the class below – the 80–93kg category – but I was still terrified of losing weight after my triple jumping experience, plus I knew that losing a few kilos would bring the majority of my strength progression to a grinding halt. And as we've already established, I was addicted to the feeling of getting stronger. It was the one factor above all that was motivating me to go to the gym six days a week while working a full-time job as a teacher (we'll come to that in the next chapter), looking after my newborn son Luca (more later!), and managing my blossoming YouTube career. So, the only option I really had was to try and fill out my class, i.e. get as close to 105kg as I possibly could. It goes without saying that if I was competing at 95kg body weight against a guy weighing 105kg, he would obviously have a distinct advantage over me. So, to make myself truly competitive in the 105kg weight class, I had to formulate a cutting-edge, sports-science-based training and diet philosophy, which I called, 'Let's Get Fucking Massive'. In short, I had to gain 10kg (just over a stone and a half) of body weight by the time the British Championships came around – about six months, to be precise. Now, I'm sure a lot of you are sat there thinking, are you joking? I could gain that in a couple of days. And I totally get it. To most people, having to gain weight would be an absolute dream. The problem for me was that I'd already been gaining weight for a couple of years and, as we've already established, metabolism is very adaptive. And seeing as my metabolism was already much faster than the average person's, I was faced with a situation where I had to eat close to 6,000 calories a day in order to gain weight.

Again, some of you might be reading this and wondering, how is this guy complaining about getting to eat loads of calories every day? That would be my fantasy! The thing is, when you *have* to eat loads of food, it's not as much fun. And even if it was, eating 6,000 calories a day for months on end absolutely sucks. Try it for a few days and you'll quickly understand what I'm talking about. As the weeks and months passed, my body weight slowly began to climb (slowly being the operative word), and as with the battle to drastically alter my body weight back in my athletics days, I started to resort to extremes. I poured olive or coconut oil into my protein shakes – literally the most calorie-dense things on the planet, with each mouthful equating to around 400 calories. (If you're wondering what the fuss is about, drink a mouthful of olive oil and then get back to me). I'd sometimes liquidise my meals so I could consume them quicker, and eating food literally became my full-time job. You know when you eat way too much and feel disgustingly full? Like you're about to throw up at any minute? I had that feeling pretty much 24/7. I began to hate food and would dread the next meal because I knew how horrible it was going to be. By the end of this period of force-feeding myself, I was throwing up pretty much every day and most meals became a battle whereby I'd frantically cram the food down my throat as fast as possible followed by a period where I'd desperately try and stop myself being sick. I would look at Sairs' comparatively tiny plates and feel envious that she could eat so little, and it got to the point where I'd genuinely forgotten what being hungry felt like.

I remember the morning before the British Champs, Sairs and I stayed at a hotel near the competition venue. I think it was an anniversary, or at least there was some kind of romantic reason behind choosing this particular hotel, and I can remember sitting with her having breakfast and having to run to the toilet to throw up. Lucky girl. I was having

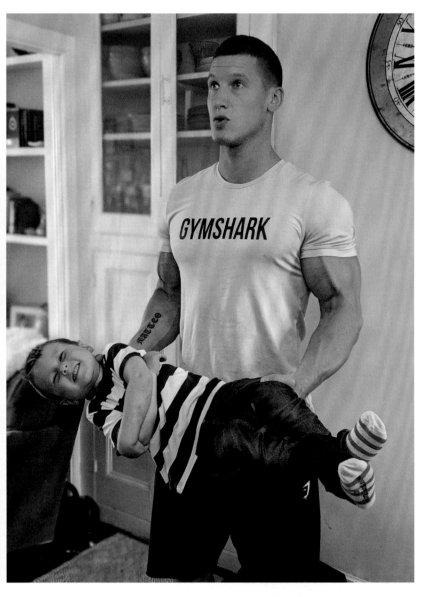

Fitness Rule No. 1: Use whatever equipment you can get your hands on.

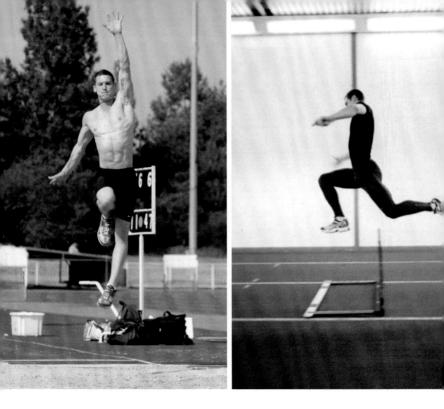

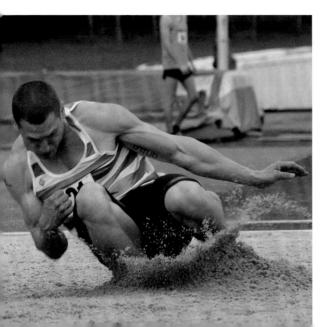

Before YouTube, PE teaching, powerlifting and bodybuilding, I competed internationally as an athlete, representing England in the triple jump.

Fun Fact: When an elite level athlete performs a triple jump, during the hop phase in particular, they load their body with up to *twenty-two times* their own body weight – so an 80kg athlete temporarily weighs in at around *1.7 tonnes*.

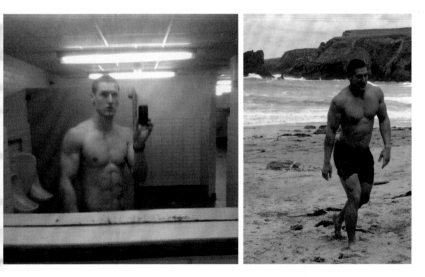

On social media, we often view images of influencers' or athletes' bodies and assume that they're healthy. In many cases, that's far from the truth. I have suffered from eating disorders, particularly when I was a triple jumper. I got into a spiral of starving myself to lose weight, and then bingeing after competitions, gaining and losing in excess of a stone in a matter of days.

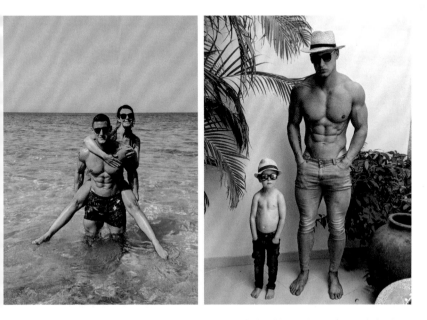

Nowadays, I'm much happier with my body and have a far healthier relationship with food. Using body weight as the barometer for the success of your diet, or the gauge with which to judge your health, is ridiculous and we need to stop doing it.

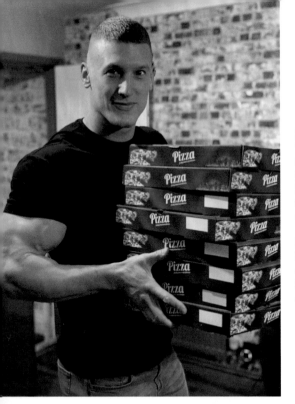

If you've watched any of my YouTube videos, you'll know that I frequently eat 'crappy' food – I always have. I truly believe any diet that says you can't have doughnuts, pizza or chocolate is doomed to failure.

I actually think it's dangerous to label any particular food as 'bad' or tell people they should avoid it at all costs. Ultimately it comes down to moderation.

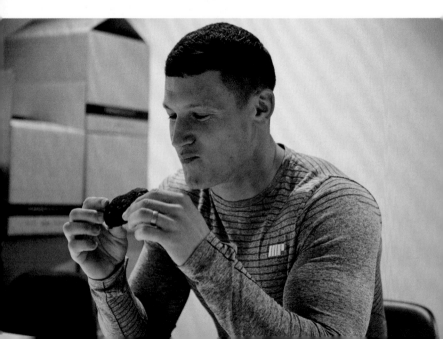

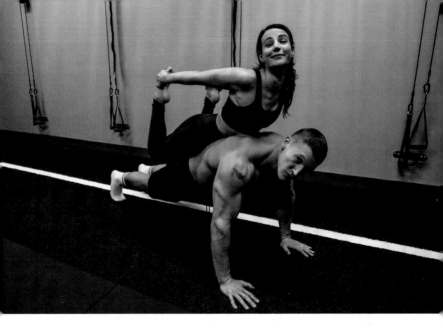

Jumping on a crash diet will result in most of your weight loss coming from water and muscle. However, by combining a sensible drop in calories with doing resistance training, you'll retain muscle mass whilst losing body fat, and look a million times better for it.

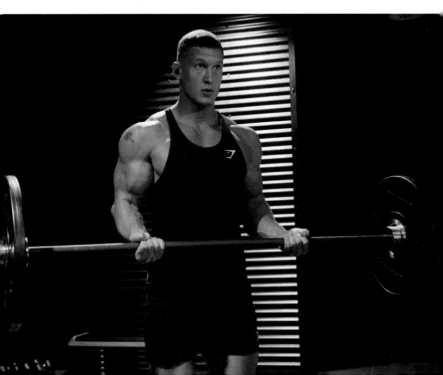

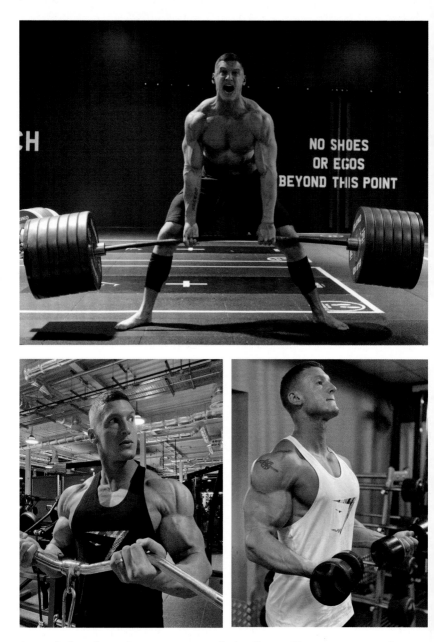

As your body evolves and improves, your standards will go up. The stronger you are, the stronger you will want to be, the faster you are, the faster you will want to be. Once you see what you can achieve, it's only natural to want to see how much further you can take it. Why wouldn't you? For most people, improving your performance and achieving your body goals will provide you with a sense of fulfilment and self-confidence.

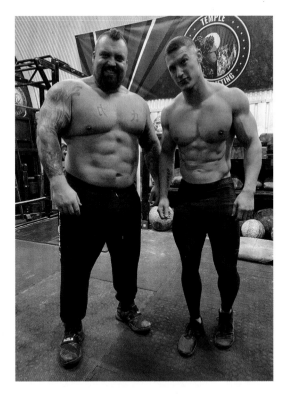

Through YouTube I've met some incredible people, like Eddie Hall, the World's Strongest Man 2017, and Ross Edgley, who, in 2018, swam 1,780 miles around Great Britain. I've also ridden a camel with my shirt off while wearing flip-flops.

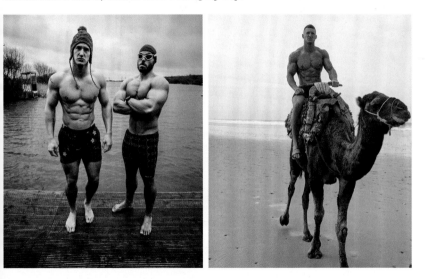

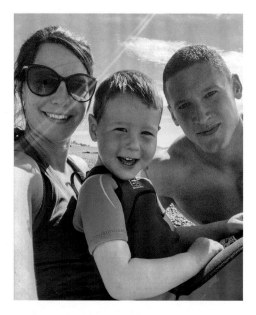

Team Morsia: me, Sairs and Luca.

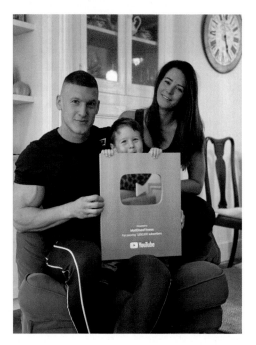

The YouTube Gold Play Button for reaching 1 million subscribers. I appreciate every single one of you.

to eat so much food that it made me sick on an almost daily basis. It was the most disgusting, horrible feeling, and just goes to show how your perception of food and eating can change. When I was trying to lose body weight in my triple jumping days, I became obsessed with food and would spend a solid part of my day fantasising about eating. But by the end of my powerlifting career, where I'd been desperately trying to bulk and gain weight, I was literally having nightmares about eating food and feeling sick. I would have paid money to have been allowed to eat nothing for a day.

What is worth stressing again here is that a lot of the bodies that look amazing on social media, the bodies you see and maybe aspire to, are built through this kind of messed-up approach to food. I've known bodybuilders who are on a 10,000-calorie a day diet and have had to employ a full-time chef because they didn't have the time to prepare that much food. At any given time, a bodybuilder is either on a bulk or a cut. The cycle starts with a bulk where you try and gain muscle through dramatically increasing your body weight, then moves into a cut (typically in the run-up to a competition) where you starve your body of calories to get as lean as possible. And this is a level of lean that the average person cannot possibly comprehend. So lean that every blood vessel in your body becomes visible through your skin, and you're so deprived of energy that you can't complete the most mundane of tasks without feeling like you're going to pass out. During the final few weeks of this type of cut, in the run-up to a bodybuilding show, these individuals are quite literally killing themselves. When you add in the impact of steroids, you can see why many of these competitors have heart attacks in their fifties. It's just not a sustainable way of life and definitely not a lifestyle that anyone should aspire to. These types of extremes are the opposite of the moderation-based approach that I constantly go on about, and I do so because I've seen both sides of the spectrum first hand and they're not pretty.

In case you're wondering, I absolutely bombed at the British Champs. That's the nature of powerlifting. There are so many variables and nuances aside from just lifting some weights, and although I was in awesome shape and the strongest I'd ever been, I accidentally ignored the judges' instructions during my bench press attempts and so was disqualified. Based on the numbers going in, I was the second-best lifter in the competition and had a very good chance of winning or at least finishing in the top two, which would have qualified me for the European Championships. But I messed up and it was all over. I was pretty distraught about it to be honest. Yet again, I'd spent six months of my life absolutely killing myself, ultimately for nothing. Or at least that's how it felt at the time. The next morning, still riding the wave of depression, I realised that I couldn't live like that any more. The thought of another prolonged period of eating loads of food genuinely scared me, and it was at that point that I decided I wasn't going to continue powerlifting. I did a couple more competitions half-heartedly, but the whole process had taken it out of me both physically and psychologically.

A week or so after the British Championships, Sairs, Luca and I went away to Malaysia for a fortnight, and over that time I ate whatever I felt like – lots of fried food and rice dishes, but only when I felt like it and I'd stop when I was full. Waking up in the morning and not having to immediately force-feed myself was one of the best feelings I've ever experienced.

On the morning of the British Championships, I weighed in at 104.5kg, but a week after our trip I was back down to 95kg. I'd lost a stone and a half, the same stone and a half I'd killed myself to gain over the previous year, and I'd done it in just under a month. Spending two weeks in a 35-degree climate, while cutting my calorie intake in half, obviously took its toll, and I definitely lost a significant amount of fat and probably a decent amount of muscle, too. But at the time, I literally couldn't care less – I'd had enough of tracking my weight and food intake to last me a lifetime. I just felt like I needed to reset my approach to food, and the best way to do that was by thinking about it as little as possible.

Over the past few years, I've accepted that I'm happy just maintaining my weight: consuming roughly the same number of calories as I burn and therefore not gaining or losing weight. It's a lot easier that way and allows me to focus on more important aspects of my life. I am still trying to get stronger because I enjoy strength training a lot more than bodybuilding, and despite the lack of weight gain, you can still increase your numbers in the gym by getting better at the skill. Some people don't realise this but getting better at executing the skill of a particular lift can account for just as much as your muscles getting bigger and stronger. Although I still want to improve my physique, I've accepted that my days of building significant amounts of muscle and getting bigger are over. I'm thirty-four now and have been lifting weights in one form or another for well over fifteen years, so it's unrealistic for me to expect to make huge changes to the way I look, particularly as I'm not prepared to manipulate my diet in the ways I was before. So, this is where I am, and this is where I expect to stay weight-wise more or less forever – 24/7, 365 days a year. If you're in a constant battle with your body weight, in either direction, you're at risking of developing an eating disorder. Obviously, if you are overweight there will have to be some level of restriction as part of achieving your goals, but I believe your perspective on that is incredibly important – it's how you label it and rationalise it that really matters, and of course, as we've discussed in great depth, how you actually execute the process.

That would've been a satisfying way to end the chapter, but before I move on I want to go back to the point I made about my preference for strength training over bodybuilding. Although some people don't realise it, there is a difference between getting stronger and getting bigger. While they are obviously connected – if you get stronger you will probably get bigger, and vice versa – it's a question of priority. The first point to make is that training for size is much more related to how you will look, as it focuses on building muscle for aesthetics, and ultimately this is a relatively subjective process. Yes, you can measure the size of your muscles with a tape measure, but that's a pretty impractical thing to do, so most people just go by the way they look in the mirror. Conversely, training for strength is completely objective: you can literally see your progress through the numbers that you're lifting, so it's much easier to know that things are going well and that you're getting better. Whenever someone asks for my advice on whether they should focus on building muscle or getting stronger, although my personal inclination is to opt for the latter, I tell them that it's personal preference and a choice they have to make for themselves.

Ultimately, they need to decide what is more important to them and what style of training they're likely to enjoy and adhere to.

From my experience, training as a bodybuilder, particularly if you're not planning on competing, is incredibly boring. I just don't get the same motivation from analysing the size of my arms and thinking, yeah, they're a bit bigger today. Don't get me wrong, I love looking muscular and my appearance is incredibly important to me. But what I love more than anything is watching the numbers I'm hitting on a particular lift increase. The gratification I derive from seeing my lifts improve over time is bordering on perverse. I find it unbelievably satisfying to see and witness that progression, and equally enjoy the challenge of setting out a training plan to help me improve further. Yes, it's also a massive buzz to look good, and ideally you want to combine both, but if you're planning to start training regularly for a long period of time (which I hope at this point you are), I just think it takes something more than how you look to keep driving you to come back.

And that brings me to the most overlooked and possibly most important training variable of all: enjoyment. With training, adherence (coming back time and time again) is *the* most important thing. If you have two individuals, one doing the perfect training programme but only sporadically, while the other is on a satisfactory training programme but turning up three times every week without fail, guess which one is going to make more progress? What really matters is consistency: doing it over and over and over again. So, if your training is boring and you find it a massive chore, you might be able to hang in there for a while, but eventually you're going to sack it off. But if your training is fun and you find it enjoyable, you're going to keep turning up each week and will even look forward to it. Burning 200 calories on a treadmill might feel like the world's most miserable task, but run around with your friends playing a game of football or rounders and you'll nail 200 calories without even thinking about it, because you're having an awesome time. I can't stress enough how important it is to find something you enjoy. Granted some elements of your training will probably be hard and you may not look forward to every session, but as long as you find the majority of your exercise (or at least the immediate aftermath of it) fun, that is everything. For me, that activity is lifting heavy weights, but it could be a spin class, going for a run, or playing a team sport like netball or basketball. Until you find your niche, keep trying new things, because discovering an activity you enjoy is more than half the battle.

I should at this point highlight the fact that focusing on your cardiovascular fitness should also form a key component of your training plan. My cardio capacity is akin to that of a ninety-five-year-old lawn bowls player, mainly because of the style of training I've done over the last few years, but it's incredibly important that you don't neglect that side of your fitness. For some people, specific cardiovascular training like running on a treadmill or riding an exercise bike seems like the absolute worst, and it's totally ok if you don't focus on it the whole time – any activity will help improve the efficiency of your cardiovascular system to an extent. *All* training, including weightlifting, will improve your heart function, prolong your life expectancy and reduce the chance of having a heart attack or stroke. But the health benefits of slotting some specific cardio training into your plan are huge, because that exercise will do all of the above to a greater extent, not to mention burn a few extra calories which will obviously help with the whole fat-loss process.

In terms of joint health and mobility there's a major misconception about weightlifting. I've lost count of the number of times I've heard someone say that lifting heavy weights is bad for your joints, and it absolutely infuriates me because, in reality, literally the opposite is true! What's bad for your joints is lifting heavy weights with bad technique, and that's where the myth comes from. People who injure themselves in the gym have almost always sustained that injury as a result of doing something incorrectly.

Someone will tell me that they did a huge deadlift and now their back is in absolute pieces but I can guarantee that their technique while executing the lift was absolute dog shit. That's the reason they've destroyed their back, not the lift itself. Puppies are cute right? Everyone loves puppies. But if I get a puppy and slap you around the face with it it's going to hurt. But that isn't the puppy's fault, it's the way I used the puppy. The puppy's still cute. That was quite a weird analogy, sorry. The point is that I am living proof that if you lift weights properly, you will strengthen your bones, joints and entire muscular structure. When you perform resistance training over time, your bone density increases, your joints get stronger, and as a result you are far less likely to get injured than the average person. And this isn't just my opinion; countless studies have proven that resistance training can drastically reduce the risk of injury, not only for professional athletes but also the average population. It all comes back to stimulus – your body will adapt to what it needs, and by lifting weights you're telling your body to get stronger, which it will. An element of moderation is also needed, however, because obviously this adaptation only goes so far. If you decide to start lifting heavy weights five hours a day, every day of your life, then there's going to be some wear and tear, and by the time you reach seventy, you're probably going to be faced with conditions such as arthritis and osteoporosis. Your goal should be to find a happy medium whereby you're training frequently, but not doing more than is needed to make progress towards your goals.

And that's a point I'm going to reiterate to end the chapter. We have all been brought up to believe that the more you do, the better you'll get. With fitness and training this has translated to going to the gym for hours on end, running miles and miles, lifting more and more weight, and pushing yourself to crazy extremes. As I said earlier, my philosophy on exercise and training is actually in stark contrast to this. I firmly believe that you should do the *least amount you possibly can* to make progress. If you can get closer to your body goals by training once a week, do it. Then, further down the line, when that's no longer enough, you can train twice a week. As humans we're impatient; we want results yesterday. It's not that I don't understand that impulse, because I really do – I'm the guy who wanted to be the strongest powerlifter in the world in the space of a few months – I'm just telling you from everything I've experienced that it's not sustainable or realistic. And actually, it can be hugely counter-productive. Sometimes it's easier said than done, but the whole tortoise and hare thing is legit, I promise.

CHAPTER SIX

WHY SOCIAL MEDIA IS RUINING
YOUR LIFE[1]

---

[1] Warning: a lot of this chapter is about me and my social media 'journey'.
But it does have a point. I promise.

So my triple jumping and powerlifting days were over. I'd spent thirteen years of my life training my nuts off, starving myself, eating until I threw up, and avoiding my friends like an absolute hermit so that I could focus on competing. Without wanting to sound like one of those bellends at an X-*Factor* audition (you know, when they play the whole sob-story video with Coldplay's 'Fix You' in the background and they tell you about how they're having to work fifteen jobs to support their dream of becoming a singer because their entire family is dead and that this is definitely their last chance to make it), it felt a bit like all of that work had essentially come to nothing. I didn't think I'd wasted that period of my life by any means, but I was definitely questioning some of the choices I'd made and wondering whether I could've done something more meaningful with my time. What I hadn't realised was that it was all preparation for the next major chapter in my life.

During the powerlifting years, I worked as a PE teacher at a local secondary school. Having spent a few years as an athletics coach in various schools across the county, the teaching job felt like a natural progression. I spent the first year completing a teacher training course while working my full-time job as a teacher, which was intense to say the least, but very efficient with my time. I was fortunate that the school's head teacher was keen to offer me the role and essentially expedite the application process for me – PE teaching spots are highly sought after (I had a number of colleagues who considered themselves PE teachers but ended up teaching maths, science or humanities), and the teacher training application process itself is a massive ball ache. If I'm being completely honest, had I not been given the opportunity to fast-track this process, I may not have embarked on the teaching career in the first place. Anyway, I taught PE for four years, and for the most part I enjoyed the job. My school was in one of the most underprivileged areas in the country and a lot of kids came from seriously challenging home environments, which was tough, but when things went well this made it all the more rewarding. Learning about some of these student's backstories was pretty heartbreaking, but PE gave them a chance to build their confidence, let off some steam and hopefully develop habits that would help them to become active, healthy adults.

There's no doubt about it, the job was eye-opening. The kids ranged from eleven to eighteen, and because of some of the behavioural issues, we had to have a very stringent behaviour policy, which was really well enforced. At the beginning, that was pretty daunting – I'd come from coaching kids who were supported by their families, wanted to be there, and who I only had a responsibility for a couple of hours a week, but this was a huge step up. In some respects, teaching PE as opposed to a more academic subject made things easier, but in other respects, it made it a million times harder. Try taking thirty rebellious teenagers outside and then giving them a javelin each and you'll see what I mean. At the beginning I had my fair share of terrible lessons, but I quickly learnt that most of the kids were looking for structure and boundaries, and that consistency was the only way to create a respectful (and productive) relationship. On occasion, I would see other teachers seemingly on the brink of a heart attack, losing all control and going absolutely nuts at the kids. For a lot of people, I think the perception is that when a child misbehaves, shouting or intimidating them is the best course of action, but my experience of teaching taught me that pretty much the opposite is true.

When it comes to kids who already have so many challenges at home, that old-school military-like approach just doesn't work. A lot of them were so desensitised to that kind of response from an adult that they'd literally laugh in your face. Through observing the best teachers, and from my own experience, I learnt that a calm, consistent approach was the best way to go. This doesn't mean I wasn't firm, because I definitely was, but there's a big difference between being firm and trying to scare a child. If a student didn't follow an instruction, rather than screaming at them, I'd simply inform them that they'd failed to follow an instruction and that they would now be subject to the behaviour policy. By repeatedly following this approach I found that even the most challenging students (who would be an absolute nightmare for other, less consistent members of staff) would behave in my lessons, and as a result the learning outcomes were achieved and I didn't experience the crippling levels of stress that others in my position did.

I'd say I became a confident teacher fairly quickly, which probably had something to do with being dropped in at the deep end, but also stemmed from my experience of coaching and personal training. Teaching is definitely one of the toughest jobs out there, and because of the ridiculous amount of red tape, you spend half your time completing pointless box-ticking exercises and form-filling, which has no direct impact on the kids; instead, I could have been observing other teachers or planning better lessons. The other major issue is how moronic the government's expectations are. They treat children as if they're robots: last year they achieved x and so next year it's going to be x + 15 per cent – as if you are magically going to lift children from generational strife in the space of twelve months. The disparity in the obstacles facing kids from different backgrounds is hardly even considered. You can't expect a child who comes into school having eaten no breakfast (because there wasn't any food at home), wearing dirty clothes (because their parents haven't bothered to wash them) and who has barely slept (because they share a room with their three siblings) to progress at the same rate as a child with loving, supportive parents and a structured home life. How could they ever compete with the standards set out for kids down the road at the grammar school? I witnessed first hand how the profession was being hollowed out, and saw a number of young, amazing teachers seek alternative careers because the pressures were unsustainable. One of my colleagues was a geography teacher, and to keep up with the targets and goals, he arrived at school every day at 5.30am and didn't leave until 8pm, when he would spend the rest of the evening marking books. He did this all term and would spend the school holidays back at school planning for the next term. And in case you're in any doubt, a teacher's salary certainly doesn't justify those kinds of hours. To be honest, it's an absolute joke.

With all of that said, I didn't leave teaching because I didn't like my job. Yes, there was a lot that frustrated me, but I enjoyed teaching PE for the most part and I was lucky enough to be part of an incredible PE department. There were about twelve PE teachers at the school and we were all mates. You could be halfway through the worst day of teaching the world has ever seen, but then you'd spend ten minutes in the PE office, have the best time and feel way better about life. That department definitely made the job considerably more enjoyable and without it I probably wouldn't have hung around for as long as I did. These days, although I spend a good amount of time travelling and meeting new people, the majority of my work involves me sat at home on my laptop, so I do definitely miss that camaraderie.

This period in my life was pretty full-on to say the least and I rarely had any downtime. As my school was an academy, the teaching day ran from 8am to 5pm, which was far from ideal. I'd typically leave the house at 7.30am, spend the day teaching, finish at 5pm, at which point I'd frantically plan the following day's lessons and head to the gym for a two-hour powerlifting session, all the while desperately trying to film a YouTube video. You see, it was around this time that I started my channel. Sairs actually suggested You-Tube. She knew that ever since I'd stopped triple jumping that lack of competition had left a void in my life. So I needed something else to put my energy into. I started filming short videos straight after work, then I'd then get home and spend the remainder of the evening editing and uploading them. After just a few videos I got hooked. Although hardly anyone was watching my channel at first, I still got a buzz out of it.

When you add in my need to eat about 300 meals a day and that I was caring for my new son Luca with Sairs, this was a fairly stressful existence. Alongside my job, during this time I was filming, editing and uploading anywhere from three to five YouTube videos a week, and I did this every week without fail for about three years, and didn't earn a penny from the videos. At the time, I probably spent twenty or thirty hours a week working on my YouTube channel without getting paid. Like literally nothing. I think this is a weird concept for most people – working a part-time job around an existing full-time job but not getting anything for it – and there were definitely times when I considered quitting. While I generally enjoyed the process, I frequently wondered whether it was all just a waste of time. It was also pretty awkward and, considering next to no one was watching my videos, walking around in public talking to a camera about my training was sometimes hard to justify, but for one reason or another I carried on. To be honest, I don't know if I ever genuinely believed it would become a full-time career, but I guess my stubbornness and constant desire to see things through kept me going, and in the end it all paid off. I can remember being sat on sixty-seven subscribers and desperately trying to hit 100. I literally planned out how I could recruit those remaining thirty-three individuals. I was over the moon with 200 views on a video, and imagined how crazy it would feel to hit 1,000. To put that into perspective, I'm currently closing in on 2 million subscribers and recently had a video hit 17 million views. That video alone earnt me more money in ad revenue than I made in an entire year of teaching. If you'd have shown me these kinds of numbers back then, I'd have lost my shit.

It's not easy trying to film YouTube videos while training – in many respects, the two are mutually incompatible, and as a result my training started to suffer. I was spending too much time trying to get a certain angle, or having to redo lifts because the shot hadn't worked or someone had walked in front of the camera. It's also worth noting that a lot of the time, the things that look 'good' on screen are not actually the most effective exercises, and I'd frequently sacrifice the quality of my session by selecting exercises based on how cool they looked on camera, rather than their actual effectiveness within a training programme. Unfortunately, this practice is widespread on social media, particularly when it comes to Instagram, where you'll see individuals in incredible shape performing the most ridiculous workouts. I can guarantee you that the workouts you often see these people post have in a lot of cases, contributed absolutely nothing to their physiques. They post them because they look good on camera and get the most likes. But the actual day-to-day training that has helped them to build the physique that you aspire to takes places behind the scenes and you'll probably never see it. It's not sexy or marketable, and so instead you'll see workouts that are essentially glorified acting.

After years of making content for no financial return, things finally started to change. Whereas initially my content was purely fitness-related, I realised that, in the grand scheme of things, fitness was a niche. If you make videos solely about training, you're only ever going to appeal to a finite number of people. The real audience was in vlogging. Vlogging essentially involves documenting your life in videos, and so, rather than just focusing on my training, I began to film other areas. I'd record what I was eating, what I was up to at home, our holidays, just the day-to-day stuff really, and as weird as I found it initially, my views started to pick up. Essentially, we are all nosy – you've only got to look at the success of reality TV shows like *Big Brother* and *I'm a Celebrity* to see how much people love watching other people do stuff.

Within the vlog content, I noticed that the food-based videos I made would perform particularly well, and this quickly became a trend in itself, whereby fitness channels started to post almost exclusively food-related content. Everywhere I looked people were doing food challenges, so I decided to get involved and ride the wave. Since I had already been eating a lot of calories to gain weight for powerlifting over the last few years, I thought filming the odd calorie challenge would probably tie in pretty well and so I started out with the 10,000-calorie challenge. I ate Krispy Kreme doughnuts, food from McDonald's and Pizza Hut – everything I could lay my hands on to get me to that 10,000-calorie mark – and to be honest, I found it fairly easy. What's more, the video blew up! Up to that point, the most viewed video on my channel had around 2,000 views, but within a month my 10,000-calorie challenge video hit 20,000 views and my subscribers started to shoot up too.

There are only two ways you can grow quickly on YouTube: firstly, you make a video with a significantly higher profile YouTuber and their viewers subsequently subscribe to your channel; or you make a viral video which blows up and results in a dramatic increase in subscribers. The 10,000-calorie challenge video did that for me, and so I made more of them. Next up was a 15,000-calorie challenge, followed by a 20,000-calorie challenge and then, finally, a 25,000-calorie challenge. Just to clarify, I ate 25,000 calories in one day. Like, what the fuck? How is that a thing. Looking back, it was quite possibly the worst thing I've ever done, and it took about a year for my gag reflex to return to normal, but in a social media sense it was incredible. The video was my first ever to reach 1 million views and ended up gaining me around 50,000 subscribers, which basically doubled my following. It was the most disgusting twenty-four hours of my life but its impact on my career was huge. Don't ask me why but people seem to love watching other people eat ridiculous amounts of food and, although afterwards I swore I'd never do another one, the video had served its purpose and my YouTube career was properly underway.

At the time, it felt amazing to see all of the hard work finally paying off, and at last I was getting some decent and sustained growth. The increase in views also meant that I started to earn some ad revenue from my videos. Basically, the incredibly annoying adverts that pop up while you're watching videos on YouTube are the means by which

YouTubers earn their money. The more views a video gets, the more money it generates. For me, this figure started very low – I think my first pay cheque from YouTube was around £50, but it soon grew and got to a point where I could see the potential for it to maybe one day become an actual job. The problem with YouTube ad revenue is that it fluctuates drastically, and this is largely out of your control. Yes, you can decide how many ads you put in your video and where you put them, but in terms of what type of ads appear, and how valuable those ads are, that's all down to YouTube. I've had months where I've had identical numbers of views, but only made half the amount of ad revenue. Factors like the time of year, the length of video, how long people watch it for and the actual content within the video all have an impact, but the bottom line is that it's very hard to predict what your income is going to be from one month to the next. On top of this, YouTube can do what they want without warning, and so relying entirely on ad revenue for your income is incredibly risky. YouTube could decide to change their algorithm overnight and your salary could instantly be cut in half. There was a great example of this in early 2020 when the platform changed the rules regarding channels designed for children, and essentially banned all ads from kid-targeted content. This meant that any creator whose content was aimed at children lost 100 per cent of their income with no warning. People who had been making thousands of pounds a month literally had their income erased in seconds. And there was no comeback, appeal or consultation process – that was it, decision made. Unlucky. It's a pretty terrifying prospect, and this is why I always advise other YouTubers to build separate revenue streams outside of views alone.

The game changer in this respect for me was when I started selling online coaching. This involved me writing training plans for clients and then keeping in touch via email in order to track their progress and make amendments to their plans. Basically, personal training but through the internet. I announced that I was offering the service in a YouTube video and within a month my income from online coaching was significantly higher than my income from ad revenue. Although this blew my mind, it also represented another huge time commitment and I would typically spend ten to twelve hours over the weekend replying to emails and writing training plans. I think it's fair to say that I didn't enjoy it as much as making videos, but the fact that I was earning money from something that I'd created myself, and had complete control over, was amazing. Shortly after this, sponsorship deals started to trickle in, and although initially this just involved companies sending me free stuff, it quickly got to a point where brands would actually pay me a salary to promote their products in my videos and on Instagram. These deals would typically come in the form of twelve-month contracts, and this, coupled with the online coaching (which was growing exponentially), offered me a security that the YouTube income hadn't.

Within a couple of months my income from my 'other job' was on a par with my teaching job. It was clear to me that this was only going to increase and, although I didn't mind teaching, I loved making YouTube videos and knew it was what I wanted to do long-term. Having had a taste of being my own boss and doing things on my own schedule, I began to resent being told what to do at school, particularly when I didn't agree with it. I'd been thinking about the possibility of quitting teaching to pursue YouTube for a little while, so Sairs and I sat down and formulated a plan. When it comes to life decisions I'm pretty aggressive, bordering on reckless, whereas Sairs is more cautious. Don't get me wrong, she's unbelievably supportive and awesome and without her input I'd probably be an alcoholic stripper in a travelling circus, so the dynamic works really well. Anyway, we decided that I'd go part time at school in order to retain an element of real security, while still building the YouTube stuff up at the same time. Initially this worked well and the extra time I gained from reducing my hours at school gave me more time to make videos, travel to events and basically improve the quality of my content across the board. The problem was that the social media stuff was growing incredibly quickly – the online coaching was booming, the sponsorship deals had grown, and the ad revenue, while volatile, was following an upward trend – and before long I was back in a position where working at school was restricting my progress elsewhere.

I had reached a point where my income from social media was now significantly higher than my teaching salary and it was clear that it was time to leave teaching altogether. At this point I should say that the school's response was amazing. The head teacher had supported me throughout the whole process, and had been incredibly accommodating when it came to putting me on reduced hours contracts, despite the difficulties this often presents with teaching. The other teachers in the PE department always offered to step in and pick up the lessons I could no longer teach, and so it's fair to say that my transition from teacher to YouTuber wouldn't have been anywhere near as smooth without those guys. Although I was incredibly excited about leaving to become a full-time YouTuber, I was definitely sad to leave that PE department behind and, as I said earlier, I still miss them today.

Aside from leaving the security of a 'normal' full-time job, the only concern I'd ever really had about becoming a full-time YouTuber was that turning my hobby into an actual job might take all the joy out of it. When you *have* to do something in order to pay the mortgage, it can alter the way you perceive it, but luckily, within a few weeks I realised that wasn't going to be the case. Quitting my day job completely changed the game for me. Psychologically, I had never devoted myself fully to YouTube; now I could think clearly about my strategy, come up with ideas and focus all of my energy into it. The quality of my content improved drastically because I was able to spend entire days filming and editing videos, and the content also improved because I was no longer restricted to filming in the evenings. These improvements were reflected in my YouTube growth, and my views and subscribers continued to climb.

Ironically, I would say the only thing that deteriorated at this time was my training. I had accepted that YouTube was now my priority, and that, coupled with a lack of direction following my retirement from powerlifting, meant that I kind of lost the desire to kill myself in the gym. I was still training four or five days a week, but if I was travelling somewhere to film some content or needed to get some training footage for a video, the quality of my session took a back seat. I started doing collaborations with other fitness YouTubers – stuff like Crossfit or random fitness challenges – and as a result my regular training would go out of the window. But I was making awesome content and that was all that mattered. Because I wasn't teaching or competing any more, it meant that I could direct all of my mad work ethic and drive into growing my channel, and I transitioned to the point where almost everything I did went into YouTube. At the time, my training was loosely bodybuilding-focused – I was trying to build muscle and develop a better physique – but I wasn't overly committed to the process and had no intention of ever competing. Training was often an afterthought; I'd just rock up to the gym and do whatever I felt like. The truth was that in becoming a professional fitness YouTuber, my actual fitness went downhill.

Typically, the second I left the teaching job, my ambition was to become the biggest YouTuber in the world, and my plan was simple: keep making viral videos. There was no, 'I'd like to gain 5,000 subscribers next year' strategy; it was more, 'How do I get to a million?' I wanted every single video I made to go viral, and I definitely became addicted to the feeling of getting loads of views and growing my following. On reflection I think I probably went a bit too far with this approach, as I became fixated with every video doing well and my channel growing super-quickly. The flip side of that was that if a video bombed, it would absolutely kill me. I would get so annoyed and bummed out about it, and would assume that there was some kind of conspiracy going on within YouTube, preventing people from watching my content.

Fast-forward a few years and, after having made over 1,300 videos, although I'm still wildly ambitious, these days I try to take a more measured approach to YouTube and social media as a whole. I understand that it's not sustainable to have my mental state so intertwined with the performance of my content, because although it's great when things are going well, when they're not, the impact on the other areas of your life are huge. To be fair, anyone who doesn't care when a video underperforms, or doesn't get excited when it does well, probably shouldn't be doing it in the first place, and I've come to realise that as long as I'm making YouTube videos, that connection will always be there to some extent. At the end of the day you can't have it both ways. Either you are invested in what you are creating and really connected to building a community (and a career and livelihood) or you're not. You either revel in the good days and take the hit when it goes badly, or you take a step back and accept that neither the highs or lows will be as extreme. For me, I'm always in, all the way. I don't do things half-heartedly, so I was always going to struggle to deal with the setbacks, and once it became my *actual* job, far more than popularity was on the line. It was my future and my family's future, and that definitely increased the pressure.

Luckily, things carried on going pretty well, but there were definitely some adjustments that came with that. The more my following grew, the more trolls were attracted to my content. I'm talking about online trolls by the way, not actual trolls. Actual trolls following me around and watching my videos would've been awesome, but the type of trolls I'm referring to are a different thing altogether. In an online sense, trolls generally take the form of fourteen-year-old pre-pubescent boys or fifty-year-old guys who live in their mum's basement. For one reason or another, these individuals thrive on making negative comments about other people's lives. Whether it's in the form of sexism, racism, homophobia or just general insults, the common goal is to incite a reaction from the general public or, ideally, the content creator themselves. I have been very fortunate to receive an overwhelmingly positive reaction to the stuff I post online, but negative comments are an inevitable part of doing what I do and something I had to grow a thicker skin to deal with. I feel like I'm immune to a lot of it now, but in the early months and years it could really get to me. Whether it was the steroid accusations or just a seemingly abstract but outrageously offensive comment, I did sometimes find it hurtful. Let's be honest here, no one likes being called an ugly c*** on a Monday morning do they? But in time you realise that the provocation is deliberate, and that these trolls are desperately looking for a reaction to gain themselves some kind of traction and attention. I've learnt that instead of being incensed and adversely affected by the toxicity, it's best to establish a level of empathy for people who literally have nothing better to do than sit at their computer insulting someone they've never met before.

I have to admit that a lot of the time I do find it pretty funny. Not that I'm laughing at a person's misfortune to be in such a bad place that they write these kinds of comments, it's just that sometimes you have to laugh at the ridiculousness of the situation and the crazy things that people come up with. How people can get so annoyed about me doing some arm curls or eating a sandwich is still beyond me. Like, calm down, mate. Go for a walk or something. I think you need to be an inherently confident person to do the job I do, otherwise it'd be a living hell at times. Imagine going to work in an office and people lining up to tell you that you're boring, your kids are ugly and they hope you get cancer. It sounds ridiculous but this is the kind of stuff you'll find plastered in comments sections across YouTube and social media as a whole, on a daily basis. Pretty messed up, right?

Social media as an industry has a reputation for being superficial, competitive and, for want of a better word, a bit bitchy. I've definitely come into contact with some absolute dicks, but I've also made some great friends in the community, too. YouTube is very hierarchical and it's funny to remember how naive I was at the beginning – I would just casually message some of the biggest social media stars to say 'Hey, do you want to do a video together'? Some of those people had 1,000 times more followers than me, but because I didn't really know what I was doing, I was always optimistic that they would get back to me and be well up for it. (That didn't happen.) Fast-forward to today and, with a combined following of over 3 million people across You-Tube and Instagram, people are now messaging *me*, asking if I want to collaborate. In fact a number of individuals with huge followings who didn't reply back in the day, have now, after seeing my growth, dropped me a message to ask if I'd be up for filming a video together. Pretty ironic, really.

Despite this school playground-like environment, I've met some incredible people doing what I do. People who have inspired me over the years and whom I admire so much, like Eddie Hall (World's Strongest Man, 2017). If a year ago you'd have said to me, who is the one person in the world you'd want to train with, I would have said Eddie Hall. Not only is he an absolute monster and one of the strongest humans to have ever lived, he's also an awesome, down-to-earth guy. With this in mind, it was fairly unbe-lievable when, a few months ago he actually messaged me and said that he'd love to do a video at some point. I ignored his message because he hasn't got as many subscribers as me, but it was cool nonetheless. That was a joke! Obviously I said yes, and we ended up doing a couple of videos together, which were not only incredibly enjoyable to make but have subsequently gone on to become two of my most viewed videos ever. And this was just one of the many amazing experiences I've got YouTube to thank for because, let's face it, as cool an individual as Eddie Hall is, he probably wouldn't have been interested in hanging out with me for a day had I not had the number of subscribers that I do.

To be honest, I don't ever really think about the fact that 2 million people subscribe to my channel. I mean *really* think about it. Obviously I'm aware of that number and I track it fairly religiously, but it's a pretty ridiculous concept. Like, 2 million people? That's absolutely nuts! I think the fact that we live in a tiny seaside town, where the majority of people are eighty years old and I'm completely shielded from any of the hype in my day-to-day life, definitely helps. Although I'm starting to get used to being approached by absolute strangers who know everything about me, it's still something of a novelty, and when I really think about it, it's quite hard to get my head around. I'll go to a fitness event and people will queue for four or five hours just to take a picture and say hello to me. Like, what the hell?! Just come and say hi next time I'm in Aldi! When you go to one of these events, though, it does make you realise that those 2 million subscribers are actual people. It's pretty cool to think that I was making videos for over three years and getting absolutely nothing from it, and now, my entire life is built around it.

I'd say that my overriding goal is to entertain people with my content, but I do try and surreptitiously inject some useful information in there too. And more and more I feel the need to call out some of the bullshit that I see elsewhere on social media. I think the biggest problem is that there are so many vulnerable people out there desperately looking for a quick fix, making them susceptible to these messages, which in a lot of cases will do more harm than good. The sad truth is that, when you are in a bad place – maybe you're heavily overweight or struggling with an eating disorder – this can lead to bad decisions, particularly if you don't know any better or someone with massive biceps and a six pack is telling you to do something. I believe the ways in which this exploitation is happening on social media in particular is fraudulent and ultimately criminal, not just morally wrong. Tea bags which promise to help you lose weight, pills to supposedly speed up your metabolism, and diet plans involving complete starvation should be banned – they're not just misleading, people are selling literal lies. And it's not just random Instagrammers you need to be wary of

– even some mainstream organisations continue to prop up a diet culture on social media that thrives by taking advantage of individuals who don't know any better. Many popular diets continue to encourage people to eat a dangerously low number of calories and it needs to stop. Sorry if I sounded a bit like Batman there but I just feel really strongly about it.

Whether it's individuals or multimillion-pound businesses, when you really analyse the plans they're selling, they're all built on the same principle: short-term results with no regard for the long-term repercussions. Sustained periods of fasting, dramatic calorie reduction and absolutely killing yourself in the gym are all unsustainable tactics which will ultimately screw you over. In two months' time, when your body has adapted to eating nothing, or training for three hours a day no longer works, you will invariably fall back into your old habits and return to square one (or in a lot of cases, return to square minus one).

So much of the language is negative. There are plans that tell you certain foods are on the 'red' list, or that eating a particular dessert means you are 'sinning'. Not only is this weird and pervy, it's also completely missing the point and basically misleading millions of people on a daily basis. Instead of solving the problem, it's actually contributing to it. As we've already established, how can certain foods be bad without context? The answer is that they can't. It simply doesn't make sense. I could 'sin' every day on some diets and still lose weight. What kind of weird diet mechanism is that? We need to look at the bigger picture and sadly on social media, you only get to see one very myopic, short-term focused vision of health and fitness.

When it comes to social media, the biggest warning I can give anyone is that you shouldn't buy in to a diet or training plan or trust someone based on the way they look. If you bought my book because you thought I had big arms, take it back right now. (No, that's a joke, don't take it back, I need the money.) The point is that someone's appearance, particularly their physique, can be incredibly misleading. I used to go to the gym with a guy who had the most amazing physique, but was an absolute moron. He literally had no idea what he was doing, and if you followed his training plan you'd get terrible results. He had a huge chest, but his exercise selection and execution when it came to training his chest was awful. How did he have such a good physique, you ask? Simple: genetics. I'll talk more about genetics and the role they play in Chapter 7, but the truth is that when it comes to building a great physique, genetics are integral. If you've been blessed in this area, you can look amazing without optimal training and diet. In fact, as this guy proved, you can look amazing with terrible training and an appalling diet.

The sad truth of social media is that, when it comes to selling training programmes or ebooks, no amount of client testimonials, years of experience or even PhDs can make up for an aesthetic physique. There are seventeen-year-old selling training plans on social media, plans which thousands of people are buying, all because they have a six pack. Some of these people have no idea what they're talking about and pretty much zero experience to draw from, but because they've done some sit-ups and have inherited decent genes from their parents, people believe in them and imagine that if they follow their plan, they will end up looking like them. Conversely, you'll have a forty-year old who's been training clients for twenty years, with a wealth of qualifications and hundreds of amazing testimonials but, because they don't quite look the part, they're just scraping a living. The truth is that when it comes to marketability and making money in the fitness industry, the most important variable by far is the way you look. I found that when I stopped training for powerlifting and focused more on aesthetics (bodybuilding-style training), I sold a lot more training plans and got more sponsorship deals. If I were to put two plans next to each other and say this one will help you squat this much weight, and the other one will help you get 'my' shredded abs, guess which one is going to sell more? It's a reflection on society really, because appearance is the barometer by which we judge everything.

I am telling you now that if you follow my advice you probably won't look like me. That's not how it works. You will however look and feel like a better version of yourself. No one can sell you a plan that will make you look exactly like them, unless that plan includes plastic surgery. We all have completely different, unique bodies. With that said, I'm acutely aware that there are probably thousands of people out there who have bought one of my plans because of how I look. They saw a picture of me on Instagram and automatically assumed I knew what I was talking about. I mean I do know what I'm talking about but they weren't to know that.

This probably isn't going to do my bottom line any good, but I'm going to say it anyway. If you're really, really struggling either mentally or physically with your fitness and nutrition, social media probably isn't the best place for you to start. But it's really important that if you are turning to social media for help with your fitness and nutrition, that you put some time into doing your research. Don't accept everything you see on social media at face value. Don't just look at one post and decide to follow that person's plan or regime. Instead, spend time watching their content, look into their experience, find out about their credentials and success stories. People on Instagram and YouTube tend to speak with authority, as if they know exactly what they're talking about, but unfortunately, that's not always the case. You don't need any qualifications to be an online coach, so before you spend your money or put yourself and your health in their hands, make sure they're a decent, knowledgeable person and have some evidence to back it up.

For me, these days my content is as much about my day-to-day life as it is about fitness. I still edit every one of my videos myself, which is fairly unusual, because most YouTubers of my size have a full-time videographer and video editor, but I'm such a control freak, I can't see myself ever handing that creative process over to someone else. A lot of the time this means putting in 16–18 hour shifts to get a video out, but I wouldn't have it any other way. I think there is this perception that YouTubers are all lazy individuals, bumming around at home and making millions in the process. That just isn't the case. As much as they may portray this amazing, care-free existence online, I haven't met any truly successful person in social media who isn't also incredibly hardworking.

One major factor which helped to reduce the workload and expedite the growth of my social media as a whole, was when Sairs joined the operation full time. She's always been an integral part of the business, mostly behind the scenes, but since quitting her job at a local primary school a couple of years ago, it has become a real family business. She does a huge amount in terms of planning, scripting, videography and photography, but she's now also a big part of the videos themselves. I think it's nice for my subscribers to see the reality of my life, particularly in terms of being a dad. When it came to including Luca in the content, we did discuss it, but, realistically, his inclusion was fairly inevitable. How can you document your life without your family in it? Particularly when you live in the same house. You can't. I mean it helps that he's an absolute legend on camera and is almost entirely responsible for my recent increase in female followers, but it wouldn't be the same without the whole family involved. I recently employed my youngest brother, who now plays a key role in running certain aspects of my fitness app, and that's just added to the family feel of the business. I absolutely love it, to be honest.

It is important to remember, however, that although people are always commenting on how much they love our family dynamic (and we are a genuinely happy, loving family), social media is just a tiny snippet of people's lives, including mine. You generally only get to see the absolute best bits, which can be incredibly misleading. I know that people see couples and families on YouTube and Instagram and assume that everything behind the scenes is perfect, but that's just not how it works. Obviously I'm not going to film Luca having a tantrum or Sairs and I falling out, because that would be weird, but that doesn't mean it doesn't happen. At the end of the day, we're all human and it would be naive to think that it's all plain sailing, particularly given the fact that we live and work together. I mean Sairs and I have an awesome relationship but try spending twenty-four hours a day with your partner (while working the same full-time job) without annoying each other. It's obviously not going to happen. Especially as I'm an absolute goon and probably incredibly irritating to be around. The point is that I know a lot of my followers have become invested in our relationship and the family as a whole and, don't get me wrong, that's awesome, but sometimes this results in people setting unrealistic expectations for how their own lives should look and, because of the skewed nature of social media, these tend to be completely unattainable. I guess what I'm trying to say is that we all have good days and we all have shit days – and no amount of followers could ever change that.

CHAPTER SEVEN

YOUR GENETICS ARE EVERYTHING

When it comes to the way you look, although your genetics aren't absolutely everything, they are 75 per cent of the equation. I know this chapter is called 'Your Genetics are Everything', so feel free to absolutely kick off about the clickbait nature of the title, but I'm a YouTuber so what do you expect? You can't buy a goldfish and then be annoyed when it starts swimming around its tank. It's a goldfish, mate.

Anyway, fish are rubbish, let's get back to genetics. They really are fundamental in determining the way you look. A lot of people don't realise this, or perhaps for people with unfortunate genetics it's just less depressing to pretend it's not the case, but it is. The places on your body where you hold the most fat, the shape and symmetry of your muscles, your ability to build muscle and lose fat in the first place, and your physical traits such as speed, strength and cardio-vascular endurance, are all limited and to an extent determined by your genes. So, to put it simply, if your parents are overweight, chances are that you'll be overweight too. Now, that's not to say that you can't override this genetic disposition and build an amazing physique, because you 100 per cent can; I've seen countless examples of individuals who've done just that. But the unfortunate truth is that it's probably going to be harder for you than it is for someone whose parents are absolute athletes.

We all know we're supposed to make the most of what we've got and play to our body's strengths. I reckon if you asked the average gym-goer, they'd be able to identify their body's assets and weaknesses without hesitation. When it comes to flaws in particular, you could probably reel off a list right now. And the pressures of social media and the crazy comparison culture that it breeds make you even more aware of all the tiny so-called flaws and imperfections you possess. Yet as we saw in Chapter 6, one of the issues with social media comparisons is that, in the majority of cases, the fitness influencers you aspire to look like they won the genetic lottery. They inherited incredible genes which gave them the ability to build muscle, maintain a relatively low level of body fat and possess a 'perfect' physique, which, realistically, the average person will never attain. It's just not a level playing field. In some ways, I think this has contributed to the idea that anyone can have an eight-pack, huge arms or gravity-defying butt cheeks, as long as they do the same amount of work that an influencer does. Most people, especially younger individuals, believe the message that they've been sold: with the right exercise and the right diet, anyone can achieve anything. But here's the harsh truth: that's a lie. You can't. You simply cannot train to get someone else's body. That's not how it works. You can drastically improve your own physique and build a body you never thought possible, but certain elements of the equation are out of your control.

What's important to understand here is the difference between a genetic disadvantage and a genetic limitation. Genetic disadvantages are areas which are going to be harder for you to conquer, but are still completely doable. For example, in the case of the individual whose parents are both overweight, that individual is going to find it harder to get really lean, but with some hard work, it's entirely possible. Nothing is stopping them. When it comes to genetic limitations, that's a different story. If you're born with super-wide hips, you can get as lean as you want, but you're never going to have a tiny waist. Your bone structure simply won't allow it. It's your skeleton and you can't change it. So spending years beating yourself up because you can't seem to get that narrow-waist, huge-bum look you've been training for just doesn't make any sense. It'd be like training to make yourself taller, and then getting upset when it didn't happen. Understanding these disadvantages and limitations, then making a realistic plan to work around them, is the key to success; it's the lack of understanding, or refusal to accept the situation, that holds so many people back.

When it comes to the way your body looks, there are three major areas which underpin your potential from a genetic perspective and we'll run through these in this chapter. When I say potential, I mean the absolute limits of your physique when starting from the baseline, square one, ground zero foundations of your body. The truth is that the vast majority of people will never train hard enough or for long enough to truly discover these limits, but they do very much exist. Once again, and it's really important that you understand this: with the right training and diet, everyone can look amazing. Everyone reading this book right now can lose fat, build muscle and feel better. That's a fact. But we all have certain limitations in terms of how far we can go, and this is something I struggled to come to terms with for years. During my triple jumping career, I ignored what was staring me in the face: I just wasn't built to be the world's best jumper. I trained for ten years but would get beaten by an athlete with just a couple of years' training.

Why? Because they were born faster than me. Or taller than me. Or just better at running and jumping than me. I still trained my nuts off and managed to drastically improve my performance over the course of my career, but I was never going to be good enough to win an Olympic medal. That was my genetic limitation.

Now when it comes to sporting performance, it's a little bit different, and in some ways, having that blind optimism probably helped me get through the tougher times, but when it comes to building your dream body, being realistic is crucial. Don't mistake *being realistic* for a lack of ambition or general pessimism, however, because that's the opposite of what I'm saying. I truly believe than anyone can build the body of their dreams if they're willing to put in the work. In fact, I know this to be the case. But if the body of your dreams involves you being a foot taller, then you need to have a word with your dreams because they're mugging you off and setting you up for a lifetime of disappointment. Fucking dreams.

Anyway, the first of the three main areas which determine the limits of your physique is your body's capacity to build muscle. Of the three, this is probably the one that you can manipulate the most, and it certainly shouldn't be used as an excuse, but simply put, some people are able to build muscle easier than others. Two people could train the same, eat the same and sleep the same, but one of them *will* build muscle faster than the other. It sucks, but it's just the way it is. However, everyone has the capacity to build muscle and so, even if it takes you longer than someone else, ultimately that's irrelevant. Like I said previously, the vast majority of people will never even get close to their genetic potential, so if you're struggling to build muscle, instead of blaming your genetics, ask yourself whether your training is good enough or whether you're eating enough food, because nine times out of ten, that's where the problem lies. When it comes to building muscle, we're all born with a combination of slow-twitch and fast-twitch muscle fibres. Slow-twitch fibres are dense with capillaries and high in myoglobin (an oxygen-binding protein), and they're more resistant to fatigue, but they don't have as much capacity for growth. Conversely, fast-twitch muscle fibres contract and grow faster, meaning that, although they fatigue at a quicker rate, they are great for growth. Some people are born with a higher than average number of fast-twitch fibres, which means that they respond more quickly and effectively to the stimulus of training, especially strength training, and can therefore get stronger and build muscle at a faster rate than other people. But, if you're not one of these individuals and it takes you a little longer to build muscle, this isn't an excuse, it's merely an inconvenience.

And if an inconvenience is going to stop you from reaching your goals, then your goals probably don't mean enough to you.

Unless you have a genetic or hormonal disorder, *everyone can build muscle*. What I find most ironic is that a lot of the physiques and bodies that people aspire to aren't even that muscular in terms of pure muscle mass. If you ask the average guy what their ideal physique looks like, it's extremely unlikely to be that of an enormous bodybuilder that you see competing at Mr Universe. In fact, in my experience, a lot of people are actually repelled by this sort of physique. In most cases, the influencer or celebrity body that people aspire to is more of a middle ground. For guys, think Daniel Craig in *Casino Royale* for example. And the funny thing is, these types of physiques don't actually require that much muscle mass to achieve and are more linked to that individual's level of body fat. Basically, being lean gives you the appearance of being more muscular, even if you don't actually have that much muscle mass. I could go on a diet and lose 10kg, half of which would be muscle, but I would actually look *more* muscular because the muscle that I do have will be that much more visible. Social media can be wildly misleading in this context, because so often you see a person's body without any perspective. The classic case is the post-workout mirror selfie, where even the most average-sized guy can position themselves relative to the camera to give the illusion that they're actually huge. I've lost count of the number of times that I've met an Instagram fitness guy who I'd assumed was massive from their pictures, only to be shocked that in real life they're actually 5'6" and weigh 11 stone. Not that there's anything wrong with being 5'6" and 11 stone, but because they're lean and they only ever post pictures of themselves on their own (or standing miles closer to the camera than everyone else – known as 'getting the angle' in the fitness world), it gives the illusion that they're huge when they're anything but. And this goes for some of the female influencers on Instagram too, who will employ tricks such as sticking their backsides out towards the camera, completely warping their physique and giving the illusion of having a bigger bum and a smaller waist. The reality is that in a lot of cases, what you're comparing yourself to just doesn't exist, at least not in the way you imagine.

I would say that up to the age of sixteen, I was a fairly skinny kid. Although I was above average in terms of being muscular, I didn't have a big frame and so, although I was always one of the fastest and strongest guys in the year at school, there were generally a few bigger kids than me. However, as I grew, I naturally developed a mesomorphic shape – that kind of narrow waist and wide shoulders.

Today, it's hard to ascertain how much of that is trained and how much is innate, because I started training from a fairly young age, but I do know that my genetics have had a massive bearing on the proportions of my body. I guess a good example would be back when I was triple jumping. Even when I'd sacked off the bodybuilding training altogether and was literally trying to lose muscle mass, I was still significantly bigger than the guys I was jumping against. I simply retained a degree of muscle mass without doing any specific bodybuilding training at all, which is obviously a genetic trait. For any younger people reading this, I really want to impress on you that you're not going to have much of an idea where your physical potential lies until you reach your early twenties, and even then, unless you've been lifting weights for a number of years, it's still a bit of a grey area. Although it's probably not what you want to hear, it's extremely rare to see a big, muscular sixteen- or seventeen-year-old. It's not that you're never going to get to that stage, it's just a case of being patient and biding your time. Yes, there's always that one massive kid at school who has a full beard and a voice like Barry White by the age of fourteen, but these people are the outliers. The reality is that, even as a super-skinny teenager, there's nothing to stop you being a big, muscular adult; you just need to be prepared to put in the work and accept that it's going to take time.

Expecting to look like a twenty-eight-year-old man who's been training for ten years when you're a teenager who only started going to the gym six months ago is only going to end in disappointment.

And for the younger guys reading this who are built like a human rake and desperately want to put on some size, I can tell you with almost complete certainty that the reason behind your ultra slim physique is down to a lack of calories. It may sound overly simple, but you need to eat more food. Back when I was teaching PE, there were kids who would work out regularly in the gym, but who would be in a constant state of confusion as to why they didn't look like Arnold Schwarzenegger. When I pressed them on their lifestyle outside of the gym, it generally involved eating a pack of Monster Munch, playing *Call of Duty* for sixteen hours and then going to bed at 3am. If you don't feed your body enough calories, no matter how much you do in the gym, you won't build muscle. It's that simple. Combine this tendency to undereat with the fact that kids typically have a faster metabolism than adults and it's not surprising that teenagers struggle to build muscle.

I should probably highlight at this point that, as a beginner, building muscle is actually a lot easier than at any other point in your life, and hypertrophy can actually take place even if the environment is less than ideal. It all comes down to the adaptation we talked about previously; in short, the point at which you're completely new to something is the point at which you can make the most progress in it. Because it's such a new stimulus, your body will absolutely lap it up and the potential for growth and change is huge. So in the initial weeks or months of your gym career, you can actually build muscle without being in a calorie surplus, but as soon as you move out of that beginner stage, that's when the environment has to be right for progress to take place.

When it comes to the way your body looks, the next major area that is determined by your genetics and which, sadly, cannot be altered outside of surgery, is the shape of your muscles. This refers to where they attach to your bones and where they sit relative to your other muscles. We've talked about the role genetics play in your ability to build *bigger* muscles, and we know this is something that you can work around, but when it comes to the actual appearance and shape of your muscles, there's not much you can do. A great example of this is your abs, or rectus abdominis if we're going in for the Latin. There are people out there with ridiculously symmetrical eight-packs. Abs so obscenely perfect that they look like they've been computer generated and can't possibly be real. You could do a million sit-ups a week and walk around with 5 per cent body fat and the chances are that your abs will never look that good. Don't get me wrong, you'd have incredibly lean and visible abs, but having eight separate sections, with your abs all equally sized and perfectly aligned across your stomach, is one in a billion genetics. It's more than just training hard and eating well, and no amount of steroids could make that happen for you. These genetic freaks were born with the capacity to have abs like this and, although they've had to work hard to unlock that underlying genetic potential, the symmetry and aesthetic appearance of their abs is something that they've been fortunate enough to inherit from their parents. Just like that kid who wins the 100m at sports day by an absolute mile, or the kid who is a foot taller than all of their mates, these individuals are genetic anomalies and therefore, when it comes to setting body goals, should probably be taken out of the equation.

Another example would be your chest or pectoral muscles. Most guys aspire to have a large, well-defined and symmetrical chest, but some are born with a gap between their pecs (simply created by the muscles attaching to the sternum at a wider distance than usual) and unfortunately, there's not much you can do about it. Again, you can build a bigger chest, you can build a stronger chest, but you'll never have a 'full' chest where your pecs appear to squash up against one another because your genetic make-up simply won't allow it. A common trait that I see a lot of women aspiring to is the 'thigh gap'. A literal gap between their thighs when standing with their legs straight and feet together. While this could potentially be achieved by having sufficiently low body fat and/or muscle mass, in most cases it's your bone structure which leads to a prominent thigh gap. If you have wider set hips (a larger gap between where your femur (thigh) bones attach to your pelvis), you will obviously find it much easier to achieve a thigh gap than someone who has narrow hips (a smaller gap between where your femurs attach to your pelvis). The point is that some individuals will find it nigh on impossible to achieve certain physical traits, despite doing all the right things when it comes to their training and diet, because their body isn't built that way.

The first thing to establish is where you are from your individual baseline perspective. That is the start line and it's something that has no bearing on any other person's start line. Your only job is to explore how you can progress from your own individual start point towards your potential limits. Of course you can use someone else's body as inspiration or motivation if that works for you, but you should never use anyone else as a yardstick against which to judge your own progress. Given everything we know about the role genetics play in a person's physique, it makes no sense to do so. It sounds cheesy and clichéd, but the only person you should be comparing yourself to is yourself. Look at where you are now and improve it. Simple. Setting goals that are dependent on variables beyond your control will only end in disappointment. I've trained with people who take bodybuilding incredibly seriously, follow a strict diet plan and still fail to achieve their goals. I remember one guy who pushed his body to a crazily low level of body fat, I'm talking 5 per cent, and yet he still didn't have particularly defined abs. There was no body fat in the way (you could literally see blood vessels running across his stomach) and he trained them a lot but his genetic make-up was such that his abs just didn't look the way he wanted them to. It was a genetic limitation and there was nothing he could do about it. Conversely, his shoulders were huge and he barely trained them! Ultimately, you are subject to the luck of the genetic draw, so figuring out what you can and can't change and then focusing your energy towards improving areas you *can* control is the only sustainable strategy.

On a personal level, I have a genetic weakness in that my overhead pressing strength is akin to that of a twelve-year old. My flat pressing strength is awesome and, at the time of writing, I've bench pressed 180kg, but when it comes to lifting things over my head, I suck. Like really bad. Now obviously, you're going to be able to lift a lot more weight in a flat press than an overhead press, but there should be a bit of a correlation there. Generally speaking, if you're good at one, you're typically good at the other, but for me this isn't the case. Instead, I have an enormous discrepancy between the two. In fact, I'm almost certain that if you were to find 1,000 people who could bench press 180kg, every single one of them would be able to overhead press more than me. Weird right?! Now, some of that relative weakness is trained, because as a powerlifter you don't press overhead, so I trained for almost two years completely neglecting overhead pressing. But I've now been training my shoulders specifically, with a good amount of overhead pressing, for the best part of three years and my strength in that area is still absolute dog shit. Like, embarrassingly bad. Surprisingly, my shoulders actually look pretty good and in a physical, aesthetic sense, people will often say they're a strong point of my physique, which is probably one of the reasons why my lack of overhead strength has never really bothered me. And while I'm on the topic of my genetic limitations, my upper chest is pretty shit too. From the front, my chest is well developed and symmetrical, but from the side, although my lower chest is fairly large, my upper chest actually lags behind quite significantly. Again, there is a small element of this stemming from my training, or rather lack of, as I don't really do much incline pressing, which would help to emphasise my upper chest. But, in reality, whether you train your chest on a flat bench or an incline bench, it doesn't make much of a difference. You cannot train your upper or lower chest in isolation, you train your chest as a whole and that's it. You can emphasise the fibres of the upper and lower portions slightly more, but it's not a significant difference, and with the amount of overall pressing training that I do and the strength I've built in that area, if my upper chest was going to grow significantly, it would've done so by now. The reality is that it's always going to be something of a weakness for me and so, instead of comparing myself to. guys with a massive upper chest and getting bummed out about it, I set myself goals which I'm actually capable of achieving and focus on doing just that.

In my opinion, the biggest issue with acceptance is the lack of knowledge people have in terms of just how big a role genetics can play in your physique. And this is also where most of the steroid accusations stem from, because, until you've met someone with a ridiculous capacity for building muscle and crazy natural muscular symmetry, you simply cannot comprehend that an individual could be so genetically fortunate. It just seems so unfair! It's often hard to fathom that someone could be that big, or that fast, or that strong, or look that good while doing the same training that you're doing. After all we're all humans so how can one person's genetic make-up or their response to training differ so much to another person's? But if you're looking for evidence of the sheer magnitude of genetic variance when it comes to physical traits, look no further than athletics. Back in 1998, Darrel Brown, a sprinter from Trinidad and Tobago, ran the 100m in 10.82 seconds. He was thirteen at the time. Thirteen. Just think about that for a second. You could take a million random adult men, put them through five years of the perfect sprint training programme, the perfect diet, perfect sleep, perfect recovery, and yet none of them would match that time. But a thirteen-year old child can do it with little to no training. If that doesn't convince you of just how powerful genetics can be, I honestly don't know what will. And there are lots of other cases of similarly gifted kids performing ridiculous feats of physical wizardry. Now, just imagine someone inheriting that level of genetic godliness for the ability to build muscle, and it's not hard to see how insane they'd look once they grew up and started training properly. The thing is that a lot of the people you follow avidly on Instagram were once one of those kids, and so, just like it'd be unrealistic to pick a random thirteen-year-old and expect them to run the 100m in 10.82 seconds, it's unrealistic for you to expect to look like your favourite Instagram fitness influencer.

Instead, it's time to tailor your goals to yourself and your own fitness stream. I get that there's a sense of enjoyment that can come from rating yourself against other people, especially if you are faster or stronger than them, or 'better' in some way. Social comparison is generally the way we evaluate our place in any society and it's natural to do it, because we are all looking for the sense of security that comes with knowing where we fit in. But when we're talking about the way your body looks, it just doesn't work that way and the sooner you realise that, the sooner you can start making progress towards a realistic goal. Remember that the most important variable when it comes to training adherence is enjoyment, and the most important thing you can do to facilitate enjoyment is to set realistic goals. And when it comes to goals relating to your body, using yourself as a barometer is the only way to make those goals realistic. Even if they aren't related to the way you look – maybe you're running a certain distance in a certain time or swimming a certain number of lengths at a certain speed or lifting at a certain weight for a certain number of reps – that is your starting point. Make a note of it. Write it down. Then make sure you beat it next week, or the week after. Just put yourself in a position where you are better than you were yesterday, and if you keep doing that over a period of weeks and months, you'll be amazed at just how far you can go.

The final area in the body vs genetics equation is your body's innate disposition for storing fat in particular areas. In simple terms, everyone stores their fat in certain places and there's nothing you can do about it. You may store fat on your stomach, your thighs, your bum, or it may be that you distribute it fairly evenly. Everybody holds fat in different areas of their body and, again, that is something you've inherited from your parents and can do little about. Now I know what you're thinking: thanks Mum and Dad, you absolute bellends. And that's fair enough. I mean I don't know your mum or dad but if they've passed down the genetics of a blobfish, I understand your frustration. However, all is not lost. Although those areas where you hold that stubborn fat aren't easy to fix, it can still be done, it's just a case of dropping your body fat that much lower. Say you've been working hard to drop your body fat, but you still have this annoying pouch of fat hanging around on your lower abs – it's simply a case of continuing to maintain a caloric deficit (eating less than you burn) in order to reduce your overall level of body fat until you get to a point that the stubborn fat is gone. Remember that losing fat should never involve starving yourself, so if getting leaner seems impossible due to your slow metabolism, it's time for a reverse diet. At the end of the day, stubborn fat is no different to other fatty tissue in terms of how it's used by the body. Ultimately, it's a source of energy, so if you get to a point where the level of fat on the rest of your body is low enough, your body will utilise that stubborn fat as energy and burn it accordingly. It's certainly going to be harder for you than for someone who doesn't have that stubborn fat on their stomach but, as with the building muscle situation, it shouldn't be used as an excuse, it's merely an inconvenience.

It's also worth bearing in mind that your body's disposition for storing fat in certain areas can work in your favour. There are women out there who are carrying a fairly high level of body fat, but because a significant amount of it is on their boobs, they still have a physique that many people would consider desirable. If those same women were to store that fat on their stomach, for example, despite having exactly the same body composition (their amount of body fat relative to muscle mass) they would no longer have that same 'desirable' physique. And that's completely out of their hands.

To use myself as an example again, I'm currently hovering around the 13–14 per cent body fat range and have been for a couple of years now (I did a Dexa body fat scan a little while back). However, despite this relatively high level of body fat in comparison to the rest of the bodybuilding world, I am incredibly fortunate in that I deposit almost none of it on my stomach. What this means is that I have very visible, defined abs at a relatively high body fat percentage. There are other individuals who'd need to get their body fat down to the sub-10 per cent range before they start to see the same level of visible abs. This is particularly true of the example I gave where the person had stubborn fat on their lower abs. Also luckily for me, the majority of my body fat is deposited on my thighs, bum and lower back, and ultimately, you don't really see those bits, which essentially creates the illusion that I am leaner than I actually am.

When it comes to those areas where you hold that stubborn fat, there are no exercises you can do to specifically target them. Doing sit-ups won't burn belly fat and doing press-ups won't burn the fat on the underside of your arms ('bingo wings'). That's not how fat loss works. You can build muscle in those areas, which will give the fat the appearance of having reduced, due to it being spread over a larger surface area, but if you're dead set on losing that body fat, you're going to have to create a caloric deficit and burn it off. Again, it comes down to genetics – if you carry fat on your stomach but not on your bum, comparing yourself negatively to someone who carries fat on their bum but not on their stomach is nonsensical. You can improve on elements of your baseline shape by reducing your body fat as a whole, but you're going to have to work that much harder than someone who has those fortuitous body fat deposit areas.

Another option is to accept your innate body shape and work within that framework. If you are a pear-shaped woman, for example, you could focus on building the best pear-shaped body in the world, rather than trying to achieve a straighter, more classically athletic physique by mimicking another woman. Ultimately, there's more to being happy and healthy than your body fat percentage.

And while we're on the topic of body shape, a growing trend within the fitness industry at the moment is training programmes geared towards people with certain body shapes or types. And just in case you're sat there thinking: 'that's an awesome idea!', it's not. It's utterly ridiculous and based on absolutely no scientific research whatsoever. The body shapes you'll see mentioned time and time again are mesomorph, endomorph and ectomorph. Within this method of categorisation, I'd fall into the mesomorph group on the grounds that I have that upside-down triangle shape (relatively narrow waist and broad shoulders) and am able to build muscle fairly quickly while not retaining much fat. An ectomorph would be naturally skinnier, struggle to retain either fat or muscle, and best suited to endurance training, whereas an endomorph would retain and build both fat and muscle easily. There are literally hundreds of fitness and diet plans tailored to these specific body classifications, but the problem is that these body types (or 'somatotypes') were defined by an American psychologist in the 1940s and represent a huge oversimplification of genetic variation. It's true to say that these characterisations are an accurate description of the way a lot of people look, but where they fall short is when they are used to determine the kind of diet or training a person should follow. Because the truth is, the mechanics of building muscle and losing fat *are the same for everyone*. And when it comes down to it, they're pretty simple. I mean, I've literally just written a book about it. And you're reading it. Awkward.

There aren't different versions of humans out there who should be doing things differently. The original somatotypes mentioned above were never validated by any controlled experiments or certified research. They were just the 'observations' of a psychologist who, by the way, also argued that the shape of your body helps to determine your personality. Endomorphs are supposedly the best company because they are round and funny. I'm not even joking. The whole thing is based on absolute pseudoscience and yet, eighty years later, it's part of the GCSE PE curriculum and you still have companies trying to sell you training and diet plans based on these archaic and ultimately irrelevant classifications.

Okay, while I understand the whole genetics thing can seem pretty depressing in a 'I have a really rubbish physical trait and there's nothing I can do about it' kinda way, I think it also has the power to be extremely liberating. What I mean by this is that, as soon as you understand and come to terms with your physical limitations, you know exactly what you *can* improve and develop and you can focus all of your energy on those areas. You can stop wasting your time on things that are out of your control and start making actual palpable progress towards your goals. That's pretty exciting right? That was a rhetorical question. It definitely is exciting. Your genetics are a fundamental part of your individual 24/7 body and their strengths and limitations are what makes you, you. If you can't love them, at least acknowledge and understand them, because they're not going anywhere.

CHAPTER EIGHT

SUPPLEMENTS ARE A WASTE OF MONEY

We've talked a lot about diet, calories, macro and micronutrients, and the importance of protein consumption, but another key area we've yet to cover, something I'm asked about hundreds of times a week, is supplements. What exactly are they? Do you need them? Should you take them? Are they dangerous? Is it weird to have a bath with my dog? I may have made the last one up, but these are some of the questions I'm asked with alarming regularity and so I think it would be remiss of me not to talk about them.

Let's start with what supplements actually are. Either natural (extracted from food) or synthetic (man-made), food or dietary supplements are macronutrients, vitamins, minerals, fatty or amino acids which you consume in powder, pill or liquid form. If you're taking cod liver oil every day, you're taking a supplement. If you have a multivitamin with your breakfast, you're taking a supplement. If you drink one of those dissolvable vitamin C tablets when you get a cold, you guessed it, you're taking a supplement. The point is that, although some people view the taking of supplements as some kind of dodgy, underground practice, it's actually incredibly widespread, and most people, at one time or another, have probably taken one. The aim of a supplement is to work alongside your normal diet to provide a nutritional or physiological effect, to support your body and help it function at its optimum level. Sounds good, right? So why, when it comes to fitness-related supplements in particular, is there such scepticism?

Firstly, I'd say that the reputation of steroids has had a huge impact on the way supplements are perceived by the general public. Back when I was triple jumping, I definitely shared that scepticism and can remember thinking that supplements were a bit sketchy. This wasn't based on any research; I think it's just the way a lot of people are raised to feel about them. For me, the whole area was a bit of a taboo and, like a lot of undereducated people, I thought that taking protein was not too far removed from taking steroids. Even these days, when protein supplements have become increasingly mainstream (a recent US report showed that 46 per cent of Americans regularly consume protein drinks, while Mintel [market researchers] found that one in four

Brits had consumed a protein supplement in the past three months), I still get messages from people concerned about the implications of taking them. I frequently hear from teenagers whose parents won't let them take whey protein because they think it's dangerous (or illegal), and it was definitely those kinds of worries, combined with a belief that I didn't really need them, that put me off when I was younger.

Now admittedly, I had a point. You don't really *need* supplements and I think it's important that I highlight this fact early on: you can make amazing progress and build an incredible body without taking supplements, particularly if your goal is to lose body fat. But even if you want to hit the gym and build muscle, supplements are still not essential. To be honest, this is a bit like saying you don't need a shovel to dig a massive hole. I mean, you definitely don't, right? You could dig it with your hands, but it's going to take fucking ages and be significantly harder. Although the research varies, it's generally accepted that, for an individual who regularly lifts weights, an intake of somewhere in the region of 1.5–2g of protein per kilogram of bodyweight is optimal each day, for building and maintaining muscle mass. To use myself as an example, I currently weigh 95kg, which means that I need around 140–200g of protein per day. Before we continue, spend the next week or so eating 200g of protein per day without taking any supplements and you'll understand where I'm coming from. It's not ideal. But by adding a scoop or two of whey protein (the most common type of protein powder, usually used to make a protein shake) to my diet each day, it immediately makes the process easier and more enjoyable. So, do I *need* supplements? No, I don't. But do they make my life easier? Yes, they definitely do.

Going back to the common misconception that whey protein is dangerous, I feel I should probably clear that one up right now. It's not. Whey protein comes from milk, the same milk that the vast majority of the population pour over their cereal every morning, so unless you have chronic kidney failure or a rare renal condition, whey protein is completely safe and absolutely fine to incorporate into your diet. There is so much misinformation out there, most of which is based on hearsay or research that has been completely misinterpreted. I used to think, well, I'm in decent shape and doing pretty well at my sport, so why bother? But when I started working at the gym after uni, I was soon surrounded by people who were regularly taking protein supplements, so it piqued my interest. Eventually I caved in, and during that last year of my athletics career, when I was throwing everything into the ring, I decided to start taking whey protein. I basically did some research and realised that for the amount of training I was doing, I was massively underconsuming protein, probably only eating half the amount I should've been. After reading one particular study on the importance of protein for strength and muscle repair, I ordered a bag of whey protein online and very quickly noticed the benefits.

During that last year of athletics, I was doing a huge amount of training volume, regularly training twice a day, and as a result I'd spend most of the time walking around in pain. That soreness was obviously a by-product of the training I was doing and, to an extent, is part and parcel of being an athlete, but as soon as I added the protein shakes to my diet, the soreness subsided. One of the hesitations I'd had about taking whey protein was that I was obviously desperate to keep my body weight down and I had visions of me drinking a protein shake and then waking up the next morning absolutely massive. I think this is a concern shared by a lot of women who exercise but are scared to supplement protein in case it makes them big and 'bulky'. That's not how it works. Although protein plays a key role in the repair and growth of muscle fibres following strenuous exercise, it's not magic. It will only contribute to muscle repair and growth according to the training that you've done. So, unless you train specifically to build muscle, it won't happen, and no amount of protein will change that. After I started drinking a couple of protein shakes a day, I didn't really gain any weight, but I did start to recover significantly quicker. Normally I would do a heavy plyometric session (loads of weird jumping stuff) and be in absolute pieces for the next few days, but as soon as I started taking protein supplements, it was a massive game changer. Now, this obvious shift was probably because my protein intake up to that point had been so low – again, whey protein isn't magic – but the added supplementation allowed me to consume a higher, more suitable amount of protein, without the added calories of eating more food, which in turn seriously expedited my recovery time. As a result, I was able to push myself harder in training which definitely had a positive impact on my performance.

Today, the whey protein industry is absolutely enormous and is forecast to reach over £10 billion by the year 2023. To put that into context, that's more than half the global market in breakfast cereal. The crazy rise in the number of protein shakes, bars and powders being sold every single day is obviously linked to the current increased focus on people's health and fitness, and we've already talked about the enormous benefits of eating a high-protein diet when it comes to losing fat. Ironically, however, if you are in calorie surplus, the chances are that you're already eating a reasonable amount of protein. It's when you drop into a calorie deficit in order to lose fat that the benefits of a higher protein diet really stand out. Funnily enough, when it comes to building muscle, I actually think that the amount of protein most bodybuilders advocate consuming is extremely overinflated. It goes back to my 'painting the house blue analogy', whereby people assume that if something is good, eating more of it is even better. Lettuce is healthy so I'm going to eat thirty-seven lettuces a day and become superhealthy. It doesn't work that way. When it comes to protein, there is a saturation point at which eating any more isn't going to yield better results. After all, the body can only repair and build muscle so quickly, and simply adding even more protein isn't going to change this. There are people out there eating 400g of protein a day, which, unless you're an absolute giant, is ridiculous. While it's not going to kill you, this level of consumption will put your body through hell and your digestive system will take an absolute hammering. As will your toilet. And the nostrils of anyone unfortunate enough to spend any time with you. Especially if, like 65 per cent of people on the planet, you have a reduced ability to digest lactose and you're pumping your body full of whey. Personally, I've never had an issue with whey protein consumption, even when I was drinking three or four protein shakes a day, but I know plenty of individuals whose stomachs tend to disagree with it in large quantities.

If you're reading this and wondering exactly how much protein you should be consuming, I'm afraid that's a bit of a 'how long is a piece of string' question. Assuming you're trying to lose fat, I'd recommend somewhere in the region of 1.5g per 1kg of body weight, and if you're happy to eat more, go for it. That means for an individual weighing 100kg, aiming to eat around 150g of protein per day. As an example of how you'd go about doing that, the following would work well:

Breakfast: Bowl of porridge with fruit and a protein shake (30–40g of protein)

Snack: 50g of nuts (15g of protein)

Lunch: Caesar salad (40–50g of protein)

Snack: Low-fat yoghurt with fruit (10g of protein)

Dinner: Salmon, potatoes and salad (40–50g of protein)

Snack: Fruit with a protein shake (20–30g) of protein

This diet would be relatively low calorie (assuming you ate sensible portions), but due to its high protein content would fill you up and reduce the chances of you wanting to eat 'crappy' food. As a result, you'd find losing fat significantly easier than someone eating a more carb-heavy, protein-sparse diet.

The point I made earlier about many women being scared to consume protein supplements is a fairly big issue, not simply because of the importance of protein in a balanced diet, but also because this is part of a wider stigma that exists within today's society. I strongly believe that many women's aversion to protein supplements folds into gendered issues surrounding training and lifting weights as a whole. It's something I find incredibly frustrating and it's also hugely detrimental to women who are trying to change their bodies and improve their health. The misconceptions stem from social messages which have subconsciously made you believe that going to the gym, lifting weights, building muscle or consuming protein are exclusively masculine pursuits and therefore inherently unfeminine. I've known women who were terrified of touching a dumbbell because they were convinced they'd automatically turn into The Incredible Hulk. They won't. You won't. The world is full of men who have spent years trying to get bigger and failed. Men, by the way, who are generally far more physiologically adept at building muscle than their female counterparts. You see, most women produce significantly lower amounts of muscle-building hormones than men and their bodies naturally sit at a higher body fat percentage, meaning visible muscle growth is more of a challenge. Of course, these are generalisations and there are exceptions, but if it were so easy to bulk up, the world would be full of massive muscular guys. And it's not. So the women worrying that drinking a protein shake or doing a few arm curls is going to dramatically change their physique need to address why they have this perspective, because, in a lot of cases, it's preventing them from reaching their fitness goals.

Another pet peeve of mine is when people, most frequently women, tell me that they want to tone muscle, not build it. I'd just like to take this opportunity to point out that 'toning muscle' isn't a thing. It doesn't exist. It's like me saying I want to drink a chair. It doesn't make any sense. A muscle is made up of lots of smaller muscle fibres and, in terms of their appearance, these fibres can get bigger or smaller. That's it. They certainly can't be 'toned'. When someone tells me that they want to 'tone up', what they actually mean is that they want to build a bit of muscle and lose a bit of fat, and both of those things will result in a person appearing to be 'more toned'. The building muscle part is key, and the only way to make that happen is to start resistance training (lifting weights).

The hugely ironic thing about this is that building muscle can actually accentuate classic femininity (if that is what you are looking for). Squats and deadlifts are great for creating a more prominent, gravity-defying bum, for example, and building a strong core with weights will create a corset of muscle which will lead to a more curvy shape. This idea that weights are going to 'turn you into a man' or that muscles will make you more masculine (with the underlying implication that it might make you less attractive to the opposite sex) is incredibly outdated and, for most women, that is just not what is going to happen. Obviously, individual women have their own body goals – some women are looking to build more of a bodybuilder physique, for example, but more often than not, the bodies women aspire to are the bodies of women who have created an ultra-strong muscular structure. Paradoxically, many of the women who tell me that they're concerned about getting too bulky go on to describe the woman they want to look like and, invariably, that woman squats, deadlifts and performs any number of other resistance exercises because that's what you need to do to get that body. For the vast, vast majority of women to get a physique that they aspire to, lifting weights is going to be integral.

Going back to supplements and protein in particular, drinking a whey protein shake works in exactly the same way for a woman as it does for a man. As we've established, protein is not some mystic concoction, it's simply a naturally occurring substance which facilitates the process of protein synthesis and with it the repair of the micro tears in your muscle fibres, caused by exercise. Contrary to what some people believe, you don't grow more muscle fibres from lifting weights; instead, the ones you already have get bigger (hypertrophy), and this is where having an adequate level of protein and amino acids available within your body is essential. And even if you're adamant that you don't want to do anything to increase your level of muscle mass and you'd rather focus on other areas of training, keeping your protein levels high is still vitally important. Say you head out for a 5k run a couple of times a week, do a few cardio sessions at your gym, or enjoy swimming regularly – all of these things still cause damage to muscle fibres, not to mention the constant wear and tear on your joints. Protein is essential for recovery and if you neglect it in your diet, not only will you experience higher levels of muscle soreness and reduced recovery, your performance during the activities themselves will suffer. My experience with low protein intake during my athletics days is evidence of this.

Another point of note is the additional challenge faced by vegetarians and, even more so, vegans, when it comes to maintaining adequate protein levels. Now we know that you can find protein from many non-animal sources (nuts, seeds, lentils, etc.), but the issue is often managing to get the full range of essential amino acids, which are crucial for muscle repair. Where meat-eaters can fairly easily find and consume all the colours of the amino acid rainbow (whey protein, for example, is a complete amino acid source), for a vegan or veggie, it's not quite as easy, because lots of non-animal protein sources only have some of the essential amino acids. If tempeh or seitan is your main protein source, for example, you're only going to get some of the amino acids needed for protein synthesis, which means that you won't recover from exercise efficiently, or build muscle optimally. In this instance, vegan protein supplements are extremely convenient, because it's hard enough for a meat-eater to get their full protein intake from food alone, let alone a vegan.

I've touched on amino acids and their importance in recovery and building muscle, and these form the basis of another popular supplement you may have heard of: BCAAs (branched-chain amino acids). BCAAs are a group of three essential amino acids – leucine, isoleucine and valine – and what makes them essential is the fact that, unlike the other amino acids, your body cannot make them and so they must be consumed through your diet. Now, BCAAs are one of the most popular, widely consumed supplements on the planet, but for most people, even serious bodybuilders, they're a complete waste of money. Let me explain why. Although these essential amino acids are crucial in muscle repair and growth, you can find them in a number of foods, such as chicken, eggs and some nuts, and so if you're eating a balanced diet, the chances are that you're already getting them. What's more, any decent whey protein supplement will also contain BCAAs, which is fairly ironic as the people who use BCAA supplements tend to buy them from the same company as they buy their whey protein. It'd be like buying bananas and then also buying a banana supplement. While it's important to note that excess consumption of BCAAs (within reason) won't do you any harm, and a lot of bodybuilders take them just to make sure they're covered, if you're on a budget I'd recommend saving your money. Even for vegans who may not be getting the same range of amino acids through their regular diet, many vegan proteins, such as pea protein for example, contain a good amount of BCAAs and so a specific BCAA supplement is unnecessary.

When it comes to which protein supplement is best, as a general rule, assuming you've chosen a reputable brand, the thing to look out for is the actual protein content. It sounds obvious, but many protein supplements contain loads of other unnecessary stuff on top of the actual protein. If one scoop of a protein powder is 25g, you should be looking for a minimum of 20g of that to be protein. Ideally more. That will ensure that you're getting the maximum amount of protein for the calories you consume through taking it. A shake made with water and a scoop of protein powder similar to that described above would usually be around 100 calories. Of course, you can add anything you want to your shake, but I would always advise that you find one that you like the taste of with just water, because if you are trying to lose fat or just monitor your calories generally, it means you have the option to keep it as streamlined as possible. Finally, it goes without saying that you need to find a protein that agrees with your stomach. As I mentioned earlier, a large portion of the population have a reduced ability to digest lactose, and if your protein upsets your digestive system, you are not going to want to take it, so it's definitely worth experimenting with a few until you find one which is sustainable for you to use in the long term.

Before we move on to other popular supplements, I want to make a quick comment on mass gainers, a protein supplement designed to help you bulk up and gain weight. These are particularly popular among skinny individuals who struggle to build muscle, and teenagers in particular are frequently lured in by the promise of gaining serious mass. I mean the product is literally called a mass gainer, so you can see why. The problem I have is that, as with BCAAs, they're basically a massive waste of money. You see, when you read the back of a bag it will tell you that a single serving contains up to 1,000 calories, which to anyone struggling to put on size is an enticing prospect, particularly considering that a serving of the whey protein supplements we talked about previously tend to be around 100 calories. So how do they do it? Have they stumbled upon some sort of wizardry? An undiscovered compound which allows them to cram an absurd number of calories into a single serving? No, they haven't. Upon further inspection, you'll see that a single serving can be anything up to 200g of powder. They've simply taken a whey protein powder, crammed it full of carbs and fats, and then advised you to drink about six scoops of it. For anyone who doesn't see the issue here, try putting six large scoops of protein powder, or any powder for that matter, into a shaker and then drinking it. You'd literally have to eat it with a spoon. It'd be absolutely horrendous, not to mention the fact that, with such a ridiculous serving size, you'd finish the entire tub in about a week. So not only is the serving suggestion completely impractical, but as a result of the extra carbs and fats (which they add to increase the overall calories), the actual protein content per scoop is significantly lower than that of a regular whey protein. Remember that protein is the element that we want in a supplement – that's the difficult bit to get in quantity through our regular diet; it's not often that someone struggles to eat carbs or fats. And if you are one of those individuals who struggles to put on weight (typically referred to as a hard gainer), you're far better off buying a high-protein content whey or pea protein, and then simply adding extra ingredients that you like, in quantities that are actually edible. Milk, banana, peanut butter, Nutella and oats are all examples of things you could add to a protein shake to get the calories up without making it ridiculously expensive and taste like absolute shit. And if you're really struggling to get calories in, you can even mix your protein powder into cakes, brownies, or other high-fat/carb/calorie foods. It's not complicated, it will cost you a fraction of the price and, crucially, it will mean that your protein intake remains nice and high.

Outside of protein, when you look along the aisles of healthfood shops or online supplements sites there is a vast, never-ending world of products geared towards fitness and body composition. Despite this, there isn't much that I'd go out of my way to recommend to the average person training to improve their health and physique. One exception to that is creatine. Although widely consumed these days, as a relatively new supplement, there is still an element of distrust when it comes to creatine. A quick Google search will yield an abundance of results alluding to the possible dangers of taking it. People will tell you it's bad for your liver or kidneys, and that it dehydrates you. I've even had people come to me who've been advised not to take it by doctors and health professionals due to the possible risks. Let's be clear here, creatine is one of the most-researched supplements out there and all the studies indicate it is safe. Anecdotal side effects reported have included damage to kidneys, heart problems, muscle cramps, diarrhea and blood sugar issues. But to repeat, these side effects have not been found in any published studies. Like any supplement you should do your own research and weigh up the pros and risks before you decide to take it, and some doctors recommend that you should only use creatine if you are healthy and don't have kidney problems.

But here's why I, and many others, believe creatine to be the most effective supplement out there. Creatine exists naturally within our bodies and, chemically speaking, it shares many similarities with amino acids. About 95 per cent of creatine is held in the muscles as phosphocreatine, a form of stored energy, which helps produce ATP (adenosine triphosphate – a high-energy molecule). ATP is known as your body's 'energy currency', and to put it simply, the more of it you have, the better your capacity to perform exercise, particularly high-intensity exercise. Now, when you take creatine, you boost your stores of phosphocreatine and in turn provide your body with more ATP. Creatine also changes a range of cellular processes, which leads to increased muscle mass, strength and recovery. For example, it increases cell hydration, which increases water content within the cells of your muscles. This literally makes your muscles bigger. In one twelve-week study of weightlifters, creatine increased muscle fibre growth two to three times more than lifting weights alone. Think about that for a second.

To reiterate, in my opinion, in terms of impact on physique and performance, creatine is the best pure supplement on the market. It's also incredibly cheap. Like, it's ridiculous. You can get six months' worth for around £10. If I was typing this on my phone I'd definitely insert a shocked face emoji at this point, or at least the creepy staring eyes one. I started taking creatine a couple of years into my powerlifting career and was astounded by the impact it had. I started taking creatine at a time when I was very aware of my strength and performance in every lift and was recording my numbers meticulously. Within a couple of weeks, I'd experienced a significant increase in my strength and some of my lifts had gone up by 5 per cent, which, for someone who had been lifting for as long as I had, was absolutely huge. I also noticed an increase in the size of my muscles and a slight increase in my body weight. Now, on the topic of body weight, some people ask me whether they should take creatine because they're dieting (as creatine hydrates your muscles cells it means you will hold more water). I just remind them that unless they are competing in a sport which requires them to sit at a certain body weight, water weight has no impact on your body composition – it's not fat you're holding on to, it's water. It's completely irrelevant. So, just for clarity, for the vast majority of people, taking creatine will make you stronger, improve your performance and work capacity, and increase the size of your muscles. There is even evidence to suggest that taking creatine helps to protect you against neurological disease. As a quick note, in terms of how much to take, despite what the container itself will tell you, 5g a day (a tiny scoop) is all you need.

While creatine represents something of a shining light within the supplement industry, another equally lucrative and possibly even more popular supplement is pre-workout. Even if you're not completely familiar with pre-workouts, you've probably heard of them in one form or another. The clue's in the name, really. It's something you take prior to your workout, and is designed to act as a stimulant to improve performance. pre-workouts come in various forms, but the common denominator is usually a shitload of caffeine. Beyond that, they can have any number of other stimulants thrown in for good measure. Why are they so popular? Because they make you feel awesome. Minutes after consuming a decent pre-workout, you'll feel more alert, energised and excited, and you'll find your performance tends to improve as a result. You can also get pre-workouts designed to boost 'pump', the natural process which occurs during resistance training when your muscles appear temporarily bigger as a result of the sheer volume of blood in them. Yet despite the fairly overwhelmingly positive effects you'll probably experience as a result of pre-workout in the short term, I'm not really an advocate of taking it, and in a lot of cases would actually advise you against doing so.

Pre-workouts can be extremely effective and, although I rarely use them, I have taken a few over the years to give me a boost prior to a big lift. The problem is that they essentially operate on a law of diminishing returns. I'm not saying that a pre-workout is unsafe per se, more that, from my experience, a lot of people become very dependent on them. You start with one scoop before your workout and you feel awesome, so you take the same every day because you want to continue feeling awesome. Why wouldn't you? The problem comes when you begin to realise that your sessions just aren't the same without it, and after a few weeks, that one scoop which had been so effective no longer works in the same way. Your body has adapted to the stimulants and your caffeine sensitivity has decreased. So, logically, your next step is to up the dosage to one and a half scoops in order to get that same outcome. I've seen individuals at competitions and events loading up on multiple scoops of pre-workout mixed with an energy drink, and yet they've told me they hardly feel a thing. The sheer amount of caffeine they are having to ingest, not to mention the abundance of other chemicals, in order to get any effect is absolutely ridiculous, and in some cases could be fatal. This is why I don't advocate regular use of pre-workouts, because I feel like it's a slippery slope. I'm not saying you should never take pre-workout – it can be an incredibly effective tool to improve the quality of your training – but I do think you should do so sporadically. Maybe you're going for a big one rep max, or you've had a really long day at work and you have a gruelling session ahead. But taking it every single day, or every single time you go to the gym will put you in a spiral that's hard to get out of.

In terms of the mainstream supplements, the ones most widely consumed and which I get asked about the most, I've definitely saved the worst until last: fat burners. What an absolute joke they are. They're so bad in fact that I'm amazed companies are even allowed to sell them. Essentially, fat burners are pills which promise to help you burn more fat. The premise is that these capsules supposedly increase your metabolism, or due to some kind of sorcery make you burn more calories while you train, therefore helping you lose fat. A lot of them claim to reduce your appetite, too. The truth is that fat burners are nothing more than glorified stimulants and are most often caffeine-based. Just like an espresso downed before a workout, caffeine will increase your body temperature, and these companies suggest that by heating your body, you will be losing more calories through thermogenesis. That's like building a sauna and calling it a fat burning chamber. I mean, technically, getting hot (or cold) in the short term will lead to you burning a slightly increased number of calories, but we're talking about negligible amounts here, and the risk of consuming the abundance of other unresearched garbage that fat burners typically contain definitely negates any possible benefit. A quick Google search will bring up numerous cases of individuals who have died as a result of taking fat burners that they've bought online. Some of the chemicals you might find in unlicensed fat-loss pills are completely toxic and anyone selling them for human consumption can be arrested. Yet desperate people will still search for them and sales from China are booming. At this point, it's worth pointing out that fat burners from trustworthy companies don't contain these toxic ingredients, but when it comes to long-term fat loss I believe they are just as ineffective. Under no circumstances would I ever advocate taking fat burners or fat-loss pills of any kind. At best they're utterly ridiculous and simply promote yet another short-term fix which is totally unsustainable in the long run, and doesn't address any of the actual problems that have caused the fat gain in the first place, and at worst they can literally kill you.

Beyond the mainstream supplements that we've just touched on, there are smaller, less exciting options such as multivitamins, cod liver oil, zinc and magnesium. I'm talking about the kinds of tablets that your mum used to give you when you were a kid. While not as impactful in the short term, there is evidence to suggest that a number of these can have health benefits. Personally, aside from the protein and creatine that we've already talked about, each day I take a multivitamin, a fish oil capsule and a glucosamine and chondroitin tablet. The multivitamin is pretty self-explanatory, the fish oil capsule has potential benefits as far as reducing the risk of heart disease, and glucosamine and chondroitin are both elements found in your cartilage (the rubber-like tissue which sits inside your joints to stop the two bones either side from scraping alongside each other). There is some evidence to suggest that taking these can help maintain healthy cartilage, and so, given my triple jumping background, I've been taking them for the best part of fifteen years. While it might be a coincidence, aside from my back, I have never had any other major injuries, which given my sports of choice is pretty unheard of. In short, if you're looking for some low-key, relatively cheap and easy supplement additions to your diet, I'd recommend all three of those.

To finish, I think it's fair to say that although there are lots of pointless, and in some cases dangerous, supplements, there are also some amazing ones which are definitely worth incorporating into your diet. With that said, 'incorporating' has to be the operative word here, and supplements should always be something that you add into an existing, balanced diet. The cherry on top. You should never use them as a replacement for elements of your diet. The clue is in the name: they are there to supplement your diet, not to substitute it. Whey protein, for example, is fantastic and something I'd definitely recommend, but you should still aim to get the majority of your protein intake through the food you eat. Supplements are just tiny pieces of a bigger puzzle. A massive puzzle in fact. Like one of those crazy ones your family gets at Christmas that take about three months to make and then right at the end you realise you've lost a piece and it ruins your life. You are not going to take a supplement and wake up the next day a different person. That's not how they work. Supplements can help improve performance and expedite the process of recovery, building muscle and getting stronger, but you still have to do the work. No supplement will do that for you.

CHAPTER NINE

MOTIVATION ISN'T A REAL THING

Throughout this book we've talked in great depth about the body and the various processes you can undergo to alter it, but we've barely touched on arguably the most important factor of all: the mind. Don't get me wrong, the mind isn't actually a thing, it's just your brain making you think and do stuff, but you know what I mean. The point is that without the right foundation, psychologically speaking, none of the other stuff matters. From the food that you're putting into your mouth, to finding acceptance and prioritising your overall health, to actually getting to the gym in the first place, where your head is at is the key to everything. I mean, unless your head is on your shoulders, you're probably dead, but figuratively speaking, your head has to be in the right place before you can move on to all the other stuff. Or does it? Maybe *exercise* is the thing that will get your head where it needs to be. I know from experience, both my own and that of the thousands of clients I've worked with over the years, that exercise can be an enormously powerful tool when it comes to mental health, and there is an abundance of research out there to back this up.

Now, before we go any further, I should probably point out that I'm not an expert in mental health. If you have a mental health issue, I'd strongly advise that you go and see a specialist. In the same way that if you broke your leg you'd probably go to the hospital, if you feel you have a psychological issue, you should seek help from someone who actually knows what they're talking about. I mean, my book's good but I'm not a wizard. And it is a serious issue. In England, women are more likely than men to experience mental health problems, and are nearly twice as likely to have anxiety disorders. Ten per cent of mothers and 6 per cent of fathers in the UK are thought to have mental health issues at some point in their lives as parents. Seeking professional help is sometimes seen as a sign of weakness, I think, particularly for men, although of course women experience this stigma too. It's believed that one in eight men have some form of mental health issue, but research shows that they frequently struggle to seek help or even talk about it. One UK study found that 28 per cent of men with mental health issues hadn't been to see anyone about it. And just in case you're unclear about the significance of this statistic, around 75 per cent of UK deaths from suicide are men; in fact it is the most common cause of death for men under the age of fifty. Think about that for a second. Not disease, or illness, or some kind of accident. The most common cause of death for young men in this country is as a result of killing themselves. If that doesn't emphasise the importance of looking after your mental health, I don't know what will. On that front, if you are experiencing suicidal thoughts, or know someone who may be in danger, please seek professional help immediately.

When you start going to the gym, or begin to implement a new approach to eating, your confidence and self-esteem may be in tatters, particularly if you've already been on a journey of endless unsuccessful short-term diets which might have made you feel like a failure. I really hope that this book will help convince you to push through the initial obstacles you'll inevitably face on the way to reaching your goals, because I genuinely believe that exercise can be the key to breaking the cycle of negativity that is limiting your happiness and success in life. Incorporating it into your lifestyle can be genuinely reformative.

One of the most important things to bear in mind when you're heading in a new direction with your health and fitness is that to get to where you want to be, you're going to need to form new habits. Nowadays, training for me is a bit like having a shower. Sometimes I can't be arsed, and other times it's inconvenient, but I'm always going to do it. It's become so ingrained in my routine that the only question is when I'm going to do it, not if. I would definitely say that I'm addicted to exercise, in that, if I don't train, I feel the absence of the feel-good endorphins which training produces. I also crave that feeling of satisfaction you get after completing a session and the positive knock-on effect it has on the rest of my day. Now, while an exercise addiction based on unhealthy body goals or overly obsessive behaviour can obviously be detrimental to both your mental and physical health, I personally believe that craving the feelings of exercise euphoria is a good thing, and an incredibly useful tool in encouraging adherence, which as I've stated previously is the most important variable when it comes to changing your lifestyle for the better. I should also point out that research has shown exercise to be an effective, though underused, treatment for mild to moderate depression, and can be one of the most accessible first options for someone who really wants to feel better about themselves.

Despite this reliance on or addiction to exercise, there are times when I don't feel like training. In fact, particularly when I'm busy, I actively feel like *not* training. I think there is this perception that people who go to the gym or who are into sport and fitness absolutely love exercise and literally jump out of their beds first thing in the morning to go and train. Generally speaking, that isn't the case. Exercising regularly isn't simply about short-term enjoyment and the benefits aren't always immediate. It's something that you build up over a period of years and your life will improve as a result. But you can build an exercise habit very quickly, in a matter of weeks in fact. You have the power to make that change in your life, and the potential benefits of doing so are so profound that it frustrates me when people deliberately choose not to. For me, there are times (quite a lot of the time actually) when the training itself is hard and not particularly enjoyable, but the fact that I've built up that habit over the last fifteen years means that I now acutely understand how I feel when I don't train, versus how I feel when I do. This knowledge pretty much forces my hand. I'm obviously going to train. It's inevitable. Why would I choose to make myself feel worse?

Although building that habit is key, it still requires nurturing and it's completely possible to fall out of the habit. I've seen so many examples of people getting to a really good place with their training and approach to food, but then a life event happens and everything goes back to square one. Maybe you've had an injury, been on holiday, had a baby, changed jobs or moved house – there are any number of potential pitfalls in life, and sometimes exercise can fall off the radar. Just like you can train yourself into the habit, you can also train yourself out of the habit, and getting back into exercise after a long break can be really, really hard. Most adults have relatively busy lives and so accommodating something extra, particularly something which can take an hour or so a day and isn't always easy to do, can be hard. My advice in these situations would be exactly the same as it is for someone starting out on day one: just do it. That's it. Don't think about it too much, don't spend hours planning it or discussing it, just go to the gym, go on a run, go for a swim, or go and play sport. Whatever it is, just *start*. And then do it again. And again. And again. And before you know it, you'll have formed a habit which, with some careful cultivation, will set you up for a longer, healthier and more enjoyable life.

Whenever I've had a break from training, the thing that always brings me back, time and time again, is the feeling of gratification that I get from exercise. Just like completing any work-related task, I find completing a training session extremely satisfying, and if I stop doing it, I miss it. Even if I don't train for a few days, I definitely notice a difference and will generally feel bummed-out and start to get agitated because my body is used to those exercise endorphins. And just to be clear, this isn't a vague, subjective emotion I'm talking about, it's an actual palpable thing. Scientists have likened the effect of endorphins on the body to that of morphine. It has an actual chemical effect on the way you feel and that will obviously have implications for all areas of your life. But aside from the chemical impact of exercise, it's the sense of achievement that I really start to miss. It has such a positive impact on my state of mind that I feel like the other elements of my life suffer without it and that makes me prioritise it every day and keeps me coming back for more.

Over the last few years, as my following on social media has grown, so too have my responsibilities, the amount of work I have on and the levels of stress and anxiety that come with it. One of the main problems is that I'm a massive control freak, and so when it comes to the four companies that I run with my wife and brother (I don't just make videos), I basically manage everything myself. Now I'm not complaining because I genuinely love my job and most days I wake up excited to get started, but at times the stress that comes with it can be overwhelming. Exercise has become something of an antidote for that noise in my head, and going to the gym has a hugely positive impact on my stress levels. There have been a few occasions when I've gone into a session feeling so stressed that it's been hard to focus, but by the end of the workout those things that had been causing me so much anguish suddenly seem less of an issue. It's not like they've disappeared, I still have deadlines and stressful situations to deal with, it's more that I feel able to rationalise each of the issues and deal with them properly without the associated negative emotion. Simply put, exercise seems to provide me with a significantly more optimistic outlook on life. That's why I'm so passionate about getting people into training and, in particular, resistance training, as I know just how profoundly positive an impact it can have on your life. And the crazy thing is that it doesn't even cost anything. You could go out for a run a few times a week with no equipment and minimal time required, and it'll make you a happier person and quite literally change your life for the better.

It's fair to say that social media has had a big impact on my mental health, but for me it's more the pressure of having to constantly create content than feeling down about some weirdo accusing me of taking steroids. I like to think that I've got a fairly good work–life balance, but it is definitely hard. What most people don't realise, particularly when it comes to being a YouTuber, is that making videos is not only enormously time-consuming and intrusive, but it also prevents you from being truly present. Despite having around 2 million subscribers and unlike any other YouTuber of my size that I know of, I still film and edit all of my own videos.

And rather than film for a couple of days and then sit down and edit the content, I like to edit a video as I make it, live. I find this makes for a better narrative, but the downside is that it takes time. On days when I'm filming, I'll typically start at 8am and be editing until 2 or 3am. And that doesn't include the hours Sairs and I spend planning the content beforehand. So, while people may see us on holiday in a video having an amazing time – and yes, obviously going away somewhere awesome is great – for me, it's not really a holiday; in fact most of the time when I go away, I end up working more than I do at home. And while I'm filming a video, that automatically takes priority and dominates my train of thought. So if we're out doing something fun, I'll spend the whole time planning the next shot and worrying about whether or not the video is good enough rather than having a good time. And that's what I mean about not really being present. Although I'm there physically, mentally speaking I'm not able to enjoy the moment for what it is because I'm 100 per cent focused on creating content. And again, I don't want you to think that I'm complaining or angling for some sympathy because I'm definitely not. I love my job and am extremely fortunate to be in the position that I am, but that doesn't make it any less stressful.

That inability to be in the moment has definitely worsened since YouTube became my full-time job, and as I've grown and improved the quality of my content, the pressure has upped slowly month on month. I'm always trying to raise the bar, so whereas a few years back I could've chucked out a mediocre YouTube video or put up a crappy Instagram post, that's not really an option anymore. I mean, it is – ultimately, I can do what I want, and I guess that's the funny thing about it all. The vast majority of the pressure I feel is self-imposed. I set myself extremely high standards and so that pressure's not going anywhere anytime soon. While these kinds of mental strains are obviously mostly felt by people who work professionally within social media, I think that so many of us can relate to it on some level. The phone is always beckoning and the standards of social media, even for the average gym-goer, are so high – the feeling that if you don't share something it is either a waste of potential content or somehow devalued as an experience because others haven't seen it, is something which has become deeply rooted in our culture. I don't have the answers, but I would say that if you're feeling that way, you're certainly not alone. It is a less desirable habit than the ones I'm encouraging you to form, and if it's something that is having a seriously negative impact on your mental well-being, it might be worth re-evaluating your priorities. Personally, I know that if it wasn't my job, I definitely wouldn't spend as much time on my phone as I do currently.

So, what about the good habits? The ones we *want* to form. Like exercising regularly, for example. Habitual behaviour is automatic and routine. You repeat it time and time again because it is, relatively speaking, easy, comfortable and rewarding. That is exactly where I am with my training. It doesn't matter how ridiculously busy things get for me, not training is simply not an option. It's just a case of moving things around sufficiently to allow it to happen, whether that's late at night, early in the morning, or while Luca has a nap in the afternoon. I know it's easy for me to say this as I have my own gym, so if I really needed to, I could get up at three in the morning and go and train, but for years I've had to make it to the gym or wherever it was that I was training (at uni it was a two-hour round trip), and I always did. Over the last ten to fifteen years, I could probably count the number of times I've missed training because I couldn't be bothered on my hands. That's less than eleven times by the way. (Unless you have extra fingers in which case you're probably really good at playing the piano. I'm not. I can play the beginning of *Mission Impossible* but then I just have to loop it over and over again in the hope that no one realises that's the only bit I know.)

You may have read that bit about me not skipping training and thought, 'Wow, you only missed training a few times in fifteen years, you must be so motivated!' Or you may have thought, 'Wow, you only missed training a few times in fifteen years, you must have no friends.' Let's assume it's the former. The truth is that I don't have some secret motivational formula, and I'm not super-motivated all the time, I just decide what I want to do and then I do it. That's it. When you actually analyse it, motivation doesn't really exist. It's just a word that people use to describe the feeling of wanting to do something. At the end of the day, if you don't do something, unless you're physically unable to do it, the reason you didn't do it was because you didn't *want* to do it. Not because you weren't *motivated* enough. Assuming you're capable of doing something, i.e. driving to the gym, if you want to do it, you will. Motivation is irrelevant.

When it comes to forming a habit, specifically the habit of exercising regularly, the initial part of this process isn't easy, and it might require some mental toughness in order to stick it out. But if you are ready to turn things around and start building good habits, I believe it is also important to identify why you haven't managed to achieve your goals up to this point. If someone says, 'I want to lose weight, but I can't do it,' ultimately they're lying. It may sound harsh but it's true. If you want to lose weight, eat less food. Be more active. No one is stopping those things from happening other than yourself. Therefore you don't actually *want* to

227

lose weight. Maybe you like the *idea* of losing weight, but actually *wanting* to do it is a different thing altogether. Perhaps you don't want to do it enough, perhaps you can't see how the benefits would outweigh the effort. Perhaps you don't feel worthy of that effort. But it boils down to a decision that *you* are making yourself, and that is something that you have to take ownership of. It's totally fine if you have other priorities in life. Maybe you're genuinely not fussed about being overweight or a bit unhealthy. That's also fine. No one has the right to tell you what you want. That's your decision and yours alone. But don't tell me that you really *want* to lose weight and then proceed to not do it. That's just annoying.

With that said, there's definitely a difference between finding the mental strength to go to the gym the first few times, and finding the resolve to make it habitual. Getting over that initial hurdle can be uncomfortable and definitely requires effort. It can be particularly hard if you've never reached a phase where your fitness routine becomes automatic and autonomous. If you haven't had that experience yet, then you don't even know it exists, or whether you will get there. But I can promise you that it does and that you will. The first few days or weeks for a beginner, particularly someone lacking in confidence, can be a fairly unenjoyable experience, but it's worth knowing that there will come a time when it's not only comfortable for you to go to the gym, but that you will do it without even thinking. It's getting through those first few sessions, getting used to the change in pace and routine until ultimately, exercise becomes habitual. It's like watching a film or reading a book that everyone has told you is awesome. You might start reading it and think that it's absolute shit, but then you stick with it and it ends up being the best thing you've ever read. If you'd given up after the first couple of pages, you'd never have got to that point. It's all about making the initial investment, so you get the fruits of your labour further down the line. At this point, I should also say that if after a few months exercise still doesn't make you feel good afterwards, or you just aren't enjoying it at all, it's probably a sign that you need to do something different. You shouldn't be killing yourself and having a horrible time without any associated enjoyment, because that is not what it's about. There is nothing sustainable about that. It's absolutely fine to hate spin classes, but only if you reap the benefits of doing them. If you hate doing them and also get nothing from them, definitely stop doing them. Try swimming, Pilates or running instead. But when you do find your thing, an activity that you either enjoy or that makes you feel amazing afterwards, stick with it and invest your time and energy into making it automatic. It'll be worth it.

Another major benefit of exercise is the impact it can have on your asleep, which also has lots of positive implications for your mental state. Throughout my adult life, I've always been capable of falling asleep at the drop of a hat; I mean, I've even been known to fall asleep in the middle of a conversation with Sairs. She loves that, by the way. But yeah, I'm a master of falling asleep quickly and I think a lot of that stems from training. At the peak of my athletics career, when I was training twice a day, I would literally sit in my car, close the door and fall asleep within seconds. Not while I was driving obviously, that'd be reckless, I mean in the gaps between my coaching sessions. It was ridiculous, but that ability to fall asleep quickly obviously stemmed from an accumulation of fatigue and my body needing to recover. Now I'm not suggesting that becoming a triple jumper and training twice a day is the solution to insomnia – there are almost certainly more convenient solutions out there – but if you are struggling with falling sleep, or finding that you regularly wake up in the night, exercise is one of the most potent ways you can treat it naturally. And even if you don't struggle with your sleep, training can still improve your ability to relax and increase the enjoyment and satisfaction that so-called 'relaxing' activities bring you. It's a simple concept really and ultimately it comes down to context. An activity such as sitting down to read a book is something which can be extremely relaxing, but if you spent days on end doing nothing but sitting down and reading, it would soon lose its relaxing qualities. That's because in order for it to be relaxing, it needs to be in contrast to something else in your life that isn't relaxing, something more stressful. Like exercise, for example. By conditioning your body to handle exercise, when you then engage in an activity which is far less strenuous such as reading a book, the feeling of relaxation will be immense because you have that context.

There's also that smug, bordering on perverse element to it – that feeling that you are justified in putting your feet up because you have just smashed a big workout and therefore 'earnt it'. For me that is one of the single best feelings going and I often envisage my body literally recovering and repairing itself as I kick back doing absolutely nothing. I think this concept can be applied to other areas of life as well. Sometimes when I go away on holiday and have a few days off training, I find I don't enjoy bumming around as much as I thought I would. Again, it comes back to that context, or in this case, lack of it. When I'm working my nuts off at home, having an hour to sit down with Sairs and watch Netflix feels amazing, but when I'm away and opportunities to relax are more forthcoming, it's just not the same. Of course, there's also a physiological element at play here, as after working or training hard, your body actually *needs* that recovery time, whereas when you haven't really done anything, that's not the case. I strongly believe that in life, you need to do the shitty, hard stuff in order to make the nice, fun stuff more enjoyable. Having that contrast in life and making yourself do things that are hard and at times uncomfortable, will make the rest of your life exponentially more enjoyable.

This is great, right? We've established that you need to exercise and it needs to become a habit. We've also established that motivation isn't really a thing and that at the end of the day it comes down to how much you want to do something. But how do you make yourself want to do it more? What can you do to make exercise and training more appealing?

One area which is absolutely fundamental to adherence is goal-setting. There is no doubt that having goals and targets to hit will make you want to exercise more. It's human nature. The key, however, is to set goals which, although exciting enough to get you to the gym, are also realistic enough that they're not going to leave you feeling like the world's biggest failure when you don't meet them. I always find the best approach to be a combination of goals covering both the short term (tomorrow, next week and next month), and the long term (next year or the year after).

When it comes to your longer-term goals, although they need to be within the realms of possibility (i.e. don't set yourself the goal of becoming a real-life Power Ranger), don't be afraid to set ambitious goals which challenge your own belief in what you're capable of. I have always been overly optimistic with my long-term goals, but have always found it to be an effective means of keeping me interested. You could set yourself the target of earning £1,000 next year, or you could set yourself the target of earning a million. Now, the latter is obviously far more challenging and it may be unrealistic, but I know which goal I'd be more willing to work hard for. At the end of the day, if the endpoint doesn't excite you, when things get tough, the chances are you'll give up. Why wouldn't you? But if that goal is something so exciting that it gives you goosebumps when you think about it, then the chances are that you'll put everything you have into achieving it.

Now, while that long-term goal is always there in the background, keeping you excited, you also need those shorter-term goals to give you something more tangible on a day-to-day basis. It's nice to feel as though you're actually progressing towards the bigger goal, and that's where having smaller, mini goals comes in. Creating a path of short-term goals means that you're constantly hitting and achieving things, and ticking steps off along the way. And who doesn't love ticking things off? No, seriously, who doesn't love that? Like I'm literally obsessed with it. Ticking things off is the best. I keep a list of all my PBs in the notes on my phone, and not just the major PBs, I mean my PBs for every single rep and set range for every single exercise I do. Remember when I said I was a bit of a Rainman? Yeah. Anyway, the point is that the feeling I get from hitting a new PB and then ticking it off and updating the numbers in that notes page is obscenely satisfying. In a year's time, or whenever you hit your massive, amazing goal, it will feel incredible, but it's the little steps along the way that keep you focused. Knowing that by the end of the week you're going to do x, and that by the end of the month you're going to do y, is a massive factor in making the optimistic long-term goals more realistic.

And for those of you who *were* in the habit of exercising but for one reason or another have fallen out of it, what now? Maybe as a result of reading the greatest fitness book ever written (I'm talking about this one by the way) you'll feel you want to get back into it but don't know how. Again, my advice would be: just do it. Don't stop to think about what you're going to do or when would be a good time to do it. Just do it. (Sorry, this is starting to sound like a Nike advert). Whether that means going for a five-minute power walk or doing a quick circuit in your front room, just do it.

People like to plan things and wait for the perfect moment, but the reality is, there is no perfect moment. There will never come a time when getting back into training is super-convenient, and actually, the longer you leave it, the harder it's going to get. Even if it sucks, even if you don't enjoy it, just do it. Because after you've done it, the next time will be easier, and the time after that will be easier again, and the time after that will be even easier, and then eventually it won't be difficult at all. You'll find yourself in a routine, exercising will be something that you don't even have to think about, something you don't have to force yourself to do because it will be easy, comfortable and rewarding. Taking those first few tentative steps is always going to be a bit of a ball ache, so take the hit and get the ball rolling. 'Oh, I won't train now because I've got a bit of a sore throat,' or 'I've got to make dinner now, so I'll think about it tomorrow.' Stop being a melt and making excuses and go and do something. Actually, finish the book first. It's taken me friggin' ages to write so it's the least you can do.

CHAPTER TEN

THIS IS IT

The final chapter. Fucking hell. I can't believe I've written an entire book. Also, I can't believe you've read an entire book written by me. Wait, you have read all of it haven't you? You better have. You can't just read random bits, it needs to be read sequentially as one unified entity. Like the Harry Potter films. You can't watch one of them in isolation. I watched *The Chamber of Secrets* a while ago and had no idea what the fuck was going on. I've said fuck three times in one paragraph now. Sorry. Although don't you think it's funny how people get offended by particular words? Like if you analyse it, isn't it strange that a combination of marks on a page can cause such offence? Why is that? I think it says more about the person getting offended than the person doing the offending. It always amuses me when people tell me I shouldn't say certain things, or act in a certain way or hold my fork in my left hand. Like, why? Why actually? Because it's just the way people do things? That definitely isn't a good enough reason for me. Doing something because it's what everyone else does shouldn't be your go-to policy. In fact, I frequently find the exact opposite yields a far better, more enjoyable outcome. Try it. Although not when it comes to actual laws. Just follow those. Like killing people is definitely bad. Don't do that.

Anyway, back to the book. Let's just get it over with yeah? So, with all of the stuff we've talked about over the course of the previous 10 million pages (give or take), you should be equipped with all the knowledge you need to start your health and fitness journey. But you might be wondering, what happens afterwards? To be honest, there is no afterwards. Ultimately, that is what this book is all about and is precisely why I didn't tell you to stop eating McDonalds. The reality is that the only way to build and maintain the body you so desperately want is to do the stuff we've discussed, forever. It's not something that you can dip your toe into for six months then go back to your old life. If you want to realise your body goals, that old life is over. It has to be, otherwise this book is no different to the thousand other shitty approaches out there already. The point is that this isn't something you need to kill yourself to achieve over the course of a few weeks or months. It's not something that you tick off on a calendar, desperately waiting for it to be over so that you can go and eat 24 Krispy Kreme doughnuts in Tesco car park at 11pm. That's not how it works and that's not sustainable. As we've discussed, that type of short-termism is exactly why fitness plans and diets fail, because people go into them with an 'I can't wait until this is over' mentality. The truth is that there is no 'over'. What you're going to do is change the way you live your life and do it forever. And the cool thing is that, after a while, it won't be something you have to consciously maintain, you'll do it because you want to and it works. Exciting, right?

That's not to say that you shouldn't strive to achieve a goal. If you follow the advice I've given you in this book, there will come a time when you'll feel absolutely great about your body, the way you look and the way you feel. But that isn't the full stop or the end of the story. It's so important to realise that your goal isn't an endpoint. An endpoint implies that the thing you were doing is finished and you're going to go back to how things were before. We don't want that. If you throw in the towel, you'll begin an inexorable regression back to where you started, which would suck. It's also crucial to understand that, despite reaching your goals, you may never get to an endpoint where you feel completely satisfied. For most people, being totally and utterly satisfied doesn't really exist. It's human nature to want more, and that's a good thing, otherwise we'd all be losers who did nothing with our lives. I know that the thought of never being truly satisfied may seem somewhat depressing, but it's actually the pursuit of satisfaction which is the fun bit. The thought of being satisfied is almost always better than the actual moment when it arrives. So, as cheesy as it sounds, this is why it's so important to live in the now and enjoy the stuff you're doing on a daily basis. I've spent so many days, weeks and months, particularly back when I was competing, just wishing the time away, ignoring the things I was doing at that moment because the big thing I had coming up (usually a competition) was going to be so amazing. I'd genuinely wish that I could just fall asleep and wake up on the day. And invariably, when that big moment came, it was never as good as I thought it was going to be. So I've learnt to appreciate the stuff I'm doing now and the stuff I'm going to be doing tomorrow, rather than always looking to the next thing. Goals are crucial and looking forward to stuff is awesome, but you can't let it consume you, because before you know it you'll be old and then you'll die and that's it.

As your body evolves and improves, your standards will go up. The stronger you are, the stronger you will want to be, the faster you are, the faster you will want to be. Once you see what you can achieve, it's only natural to want to see how much further you can take it. Why wouldn't you? But you're probably never going to say: that's it, I've peaked, I'm done, I look amazing, my performance is amazing, my work here is over. For most people, improving your performance and achieving your body goals will provide you with a sense of fulfilment and self-confidence, but once that feeling fades, which it will, it's something you'll miss and so new goals need to be set. You can equate those shifting standards to lifting weights. When I was a kid, the idea of lifting 100kg seemed like the most ridiculous thing. How could anyone ever lift that kind of weight off the ground? But then I did, and as soon as I'd lifted it a few times, it became the norm, and my expectations of myself changed. Before I knew it, I was imagining lifting 150kg, and then 200kg, and then 300kg, and my whole frame of reference continued to move upwards.

It's also important to remember that, when it comes to your performance and appearance, your body needs sufficient stimulus to continue looking good and performing well. It won't do it without you holding up your end of the bargain. If you achieve your goals and then take your foot off the pedal, eventually you're going to regress. Even if you maintain the level of work you've been doing to get to that point, it's not enough. Remember that your body is extremely adept at adaptation and it craves that equilibrium, so the first sign it gets that you're not interested in pushing it anymore, it'll stop progressing and, in time, actually start to go backwards. I'm not saying that you'll have to continue increasing the workload until you hit the age of sixty and you're training for ten hours a day, but you need to keep changing the stimulus and make it more challenging in some way. And not just for your body, but also for your mind. How boring would it be to just keep doing the same thing for months on end? I know it definitely wouldn't be enough to keep me going to the gym.

I'm now at the point in my training where progress is slow. That's inevitable. As a beginner, you can progress at a crazy rate, but once you reach a point where you've been training at a high level for so long, things are much less changeable. Unless I was to commit to a drastic drop or increase in calories, my physique isn't going to change that much, and I've accepted this fact. The reality is that, after years of training, my body is so conditioned to the stimulus of resistance training that it no longer has the same effect. Also, I've already built a large portion of the muscle mass that I'm capable of building, and so, my ability to build additional muscle mass has diminished compared to when I first started out all those years ago. But rather than cry about the fact that I now need to train hard four to five days a week just to *maintain* my physique, I've shifted my goals back towards performance. Building muscle takes a long time, and the longer you train for, the harder it is to accomplish. But in terms of performance and learning skills, you can continue improving forever. Despite the years I've spent lifting weights, my lifts continue to reach unprecedented levels and my squat, bench and deadlift are currently the best they have ever been. My size, level of body fat and overall appearance has remained steady for the last few years, but my performance is getting better and better, and that's something I can continue to work on for many years to come. That's the great thing about performance, you can always get better at a skill. Whether that's doing a squat or kicking a football, perfecting your golf swing or throwing a basketball into a hoop, there will always be room for improvement, and I find that really exciting.

When it comes to your diet, don't panic, I'm not about to tell you to continue counting your calories forever. Instead, there'll come a time in the not too distant future when you're so good at estimating how many calories (and how much protein) is in different foods that it's no longer necessary. It'll become an intuitive process, and as a result, life will get easier. The reality is that most people tend to eat the same stuff day-to-day anyway, so it really won't take that long to learn what's in the foods you eat and how it all fits into your overall plan. Although essential in the initial stages of this process, in the long term I don't think that counting calories is healthy. Not only is it a bit of a pain, but if you're not careful, it can lead to an eating disorder. If you track every mouthful you eat, over time it's almost impossible not to get a bit obsessed with it, and that can lead to overly controlled, disordered eating. For a short time, calorie counting is really instructive and informative and will make you look at what you're consuming very differently. But before you know it, you'll be able to stop reading the labels on stuff and emergency googling the nutritional values of different foods. At this point you'll find the whole process much easier. The only exception to this rule is if you embark on a reverse diet. For this to work properly, every single calorie is key, because you're working with very fine margins and so an extra 100 calories here or there does make a difference.

When you do reach the point where you intuitively know what and how much to eat, you'll be able to relax somewhat when it comes to your food choices and calories as a whole. I mean, I think you should always be relaxed when it comes to food consumption, because at the end of the day, no one is making you eat stuff – you're in complete control of that, but with that experience will come an ability to auto-regulate your diet from day to day. So if you eat out with friends for a few days running, or just have a day when you feel like shit and end up eating more than you planned, you'll instinctively understand the need to drop your calories a little over the next few days to accommodate this accordingly. Conversely, if you have a few days where you're super-busy at work and miss a couple of meals, you can easily bump up your calories for a day or so to ensure you don't lose any hard-earned muscle mass. It's key to remember, however, that this is a gradual process of levelling things out and not a yo-yo approach. It's not a case of going nuts and eating 10,000 calories of junk food followed by a couple of days of absolute starvation to punish yourself and make up for it. It's simply a logical process of dropping your calories slightly over the course of a few days until the extra calories you consumed previously have been accounted for. Easy. There shouldn't be any guilt involved, it's just a long-term, sustainable approach to life.

You'll also develop a good understanding of the way you look, the way you're performing in the gym (or whatever form of exercise you choose to do), and possibly your weight on the scales, although remember the absolute plethora of variables involved when it comes to body weight. This can then be factored into that auto-regulation of your diet I just mentioned, so if you notice a pattern of weight gain over a few weeks, if your clothes are feeling a little tight or you can see an increase in fat on a particular part of your body, all you need to do is rein in your eating a bit. That's assuming you're looking to lose or maintain body fat obviously. Conversely, if you're dropping weight and you don't want to be, you simply eat a little bit more. It's so painstakingly simple that people don't believe it, but that's honestly as deep as it gets.

That's where I'm at now. I've become very good at estimating roughly how many calories and how much protein is in different types of food, so I no longer have to consciously think about it every time I eat. But that takes time and practice, like any skill. While I don't think about it too deeply, from time to time I have to eat a little bit more or a little bit less than I might want to, to get back to where I need to be, but it's not stressful or uncomfortable, it's just a simple readjustment that requires minimal effort on my part. Now that I'm eating in a sustainable and relatively healthy way (lots of fruit and vegetables, coupled with fibre and protein-dense foods, and of course some junk because it tastes nice), I don't ever have the desire to go nuts and eat 10,000 calories; that urge just isn't there any more. As long as you don't arbitrarily ban things or demonise certain food groups, you won't develop those ridiculous cravings and that will make life so much more enjoyable. I'm aware that this may feel incredibly unrealistic to you right now, because maybe you've been dieting for years or perhaps you've inherited the metabolism of a slug. You may have been through years of disordered eating and the idea of not having to think about every little thing you put into your mouth seems incomprehensible. But if you commit to the lessons in this book, and you're patient, there's a great chance you *will* get to a point where you are able to consume a good number of calories without any guilt or adverse effects. The time *will* come when you're able to switch off and have a more relaxed attitude to food, all while building and maintaining the body of your dreams. But getting to that point isn't easy and you'll have to work to get there.

Now, you may be thinking that this all sounds like a lot of hard work, and maybe you're not convinced that you have the drive or dedication to do it 'this way'. What I want to impress upon you here for the last time is that *this* is the *only* way. I haven't come up with anything wildly revolutionary, it's not a new-age, undiscovered approach to diet and training, I'm not sat here waiting for my Nobel Prize. This is just how the body works. If you don't like it or you think it's not for you, that's absolutely fine, but if you genuinely want to change your body for the better, you don't have any other option. You're stuck with me. Sorry. This is awkward now isn't it? Like when you have an argument with someone in a car but then you have to sit next to them for an hour while you circumnavigate the M25. Anyway, as

I was saying, I can totally see how tempting it is to believe that there must something easier out there, something quicker, but I'm afraid that's not the case. It doesn't exist. That's assuming you want to make a permanent change that is. I mean, if you just want to change your body for a few weeks there's loads of easier shit you can do. Just scroll through the Instagram fitness explore page for ten minutes and you'll be good to go.

Before I go, I want to leave you with another one of my classic analogies, because this is my book and I can do what I want. Imagine you're driving your car and the engine starts smoking. Shit right? Not ideal. Anyway, you carry on because you're in a rush and soon the car completely packs up. The engine stops working entirely and you're basically screwed. But fortunately you're on a massive hill, and you're at the top of it. Yes! This is amazing, right? Now you can just roll your car down the hill and cruise along for another mile or so. Absolute result. The problem is, of course, that as soon as you get to the bottom of the hill and you lose that momentum, your car is going to stop and it's still broken. In fact, you've probably made it worse by rolling it down a massive hill, you moron. This is exactly what millions of people across the world are choosing to do on a daily basis. They're choosing to follow a short-term approach to diet and training with no regard for the longer-term implications. It may take longer and be a massive pain in the arse, but by taking your car to the garage you can have it repaired and learn what you need to do to prevent it from breaking down again.

If you picked this book up because you were thinking 'New year, new me,' or 'I need a summer holiday body,' you're going to be feeling a little short-changed right now. Don't worry, I'm sure Penguin will sort out a refund or something (actually, my editor says that's not going to happen). In the meantime, just think about the crash diet or six-week training programme that you thought you were about to embark on. Can you imagine yourself doing it every day for the rest of your life? If the answer to that question is no, then you're wasting your time. If what you are doing is whimsical, or you're just jumping on the bandwagon to change your body in a matter of weeks, it's not going to work for long. Soon the momentum you got from rolling down the hill will run out and your car will still be broken. Nothing's actually changed.

And even if you do completely understand what I'm on about, the chances are that when you're done reading, you'll still put the book down and go back to your regular life. That's just what people do. We love comfort zones. Doing what we've always done is extremely comfortable. And that's what generally separates the people who are successful and achieve stuff, from the people who don't. They're willing to step out of their comfort zones and continue doing it until they get what they want. And remember – there will never be a 'right time' to start doing this. You're not going to wake up and think 'This is the day! Everything has fallen into place and this is the moment that I start my journey to a better and healthier life.' That's not going to happen. What will happen is that you'll wait until tomorrow, and then the day after, and before you know it you'll be older and have even more responsibilities that get in the way. Then you'll have that same moment of realisation that you're not really happy with your body and you should really do something about it, and the cycle will continue. So why don't you stop pretending that you're too busy to do anything about it and actually do something? Like literally get up now and do something. Go for a run. Or a hard walk. Or a bike ride. Or go to a gym. Or figure out how you're going to change your diet and start losing body fat. But please, don't read this whole book and not actually do anything about it. You have the power right now, exactly as you are, to change your life and make your existence exponentially more enjoyable. You can literally make your life better. Why would you choose not to do that? Because it's a bit uncomfortable? Are you joking?

I'm going to finish with a quick story about someone called Amy Purdy. She's an American snowboarder who, at the age of nineteen, contracted bacterial meningitis and had to have both of her legs amputated below the knee. She lost both kidneys, had a transplant and her spleen was removed. Doctors gave her a 2 per cent chance of survival. She survived. Then, because there weren't any prosthetics versatile enough to allow her to snowboard, she built her own and went on to win the Para-Snowboarding World Championships. You're telling me that losing weight or getting a better body is too hard, but Amy Purdy can literally build her own legs and become a world champion snowboarder? I'm not buying it, mate. Decide what you really want, set yourself a goal, make a plan of how you're going to reach it and then go out and do it.

Thanks for reading! If you enjoyed the book, feel free to follow me on YouTube or Instagram @MattDoesFitness.

REFERENCES

p. 35 TheTimes.co.uk, ' Impossible goals: the new demands on male physique': https://www.thetimes.co.uk/edition/news/impossible-goals-the-new-demands-on-male-physique-gr6hx2dln

p. 40 Gerald T Mangine, Jay R Hoffman, Adam M Gonzalez, Jeremy R Townsend, Adam J Wells, Adam R Jajtner, Kyle S Beyer, Carleigh H Boone, Amelia A Miramonti, Ran Wang, Michael B LaMonica, David H Fukuda, Nicholas A Ratamess, and Jeffrey R Stout, 'Building muscle increases metabolism: The effect of training volume and intensity on improvements in muscular strength and size in resistance-trained men': https://www.ncbi.nlm.nih.gov/pmc/articles/PMC4562558/

p. 53 Nicolas D. Knuth, Darcy L. Johannsen, Robyn A. Tamboli, Pamela A. Marks-Shulman, Robert Huizenga, Kong Y. Chen, Naji N. Abumrad, Eric Ravussin, and Kevin D. Hall, 'Metabolism adaptions: Metabolic adaptation following massive weight loss is related to the degree of energy imbalance and changes in circulating leptin': https://www.ncbi.nlm.nih.gov/pmc/articles/PMC4236233/

p. 55 David E Cummings , David S Weigle, R Scott Frayo, Patricia A Breen, Marina K Ma, E Patchen Dellinger, Jonathan Q Purnell, 'Plasma ghrelin levels after diet-induced weight loss or gastric bypass surgery': https://pubmed.ncbi.nlm.nih.gov/12023994/

p. 56 Dominik H Pesta and Varman T Samuel, 'Thermogenic and satiating effect of protein: A high-protein diet for reducing body fat: mechanisms and possible caveats': https://www.ncbi.nlm.nih.gov/pmc/articles/PMC4258944/

p. 66 UCLA Newsroom, 'Regaining weight: Dieting does not work, UCLA researchers report' https://newsroom.ucla.edu/releases/Dieting-Does-Not-Work-UCLA-Researchers-7832

p. 70 Frank M. Sacks, M.D., George A. Bray, M.D., Vincent J. Carey, Ph.D., Steven R. Smith, M.D., Donna H. Ryan, M.D., Stephen D. Anton, Ph.D., Katherine McManus, M.S., R.D., Catherine M. Champagne, Ph.D., Louise M. Bishop, M.S., R.D., Nancy Laranjo, B.A., Meryl S. Leboff, M.D., Jennifer C. Rood, Ph.D., Lilian de Jonge, Ph.D., Frank L. Greenway, M.D., Catherine M. Loria, Ph.D., Eva Obarzanek, Ph.D., and Donald A. Williamson, Ph.D., 'Carbs and fats don't matter: Comparison of Weight-Loss Diets with Different Compositions of Fat, Protein, and Carbohydrates': https://www.ncbi.nlm.nih.gov/pmc/articles/PMC2763382/#t=articleBackground

p. 73 Jameason D Cameron, Marie-Josée Cyr, Eric Doucet, 'Increased meal frequency does not promote greater weight loss in subjects who were pre-scribed an 8-week equi-energetic energy-restricted diet': https://pubmed.ncbi.nlm.nih.gov/19943985/

p. 74 CNN.com, ' Twinkie diet helps nutrition professor lose 27 pounds': http://edition.cnn.com/2010/HEALTH/11/08/twinkie.diet.professor/index.html

p. 75 Diabetes.org.uk, 'Sugar and diabetes': https://www.diabetes.org.uk/Guide-to-diabetes/Enjoy-food/Eating-with-diabetes/Diabetes-food-myths/Myth-sugar-causes-diabetes

p. 75 Jung Eun Kim and Wayne W. Campbell, 'Dietary Cholesterol Contained in Whole Eggs Is Not Well Absorbed and Does Not Acutely Affect Plasma Total Cholesterol Concentration in Men and Women: Results from 2 Randomized Controlled Crossover Studies': https://www.ncbi.nlm.nih.gov/pmc/articles/PMC6165023/#:~:text=In%20conclusion%2C%20results%20from%20these,increase%20plasma%20total%20cholesterol%20concentration

pp. 79–80 ' TheConversation.com, 'Faster, higher, stronger: science shows why triple jumpers may be the ultimate Olympians': https://theconversation.com/faster-higher-stronger-science-shows-why-triple-jumpers-may-be-the-ultimate-olympians-63975

pp. 79–80 Thomas W. Kaminski, PhD, ATC, FNATA, FACSM; Jay Hertel, PhD, ATC, FNATA, FACSM; Ned Amendola, MD; Carrie L. Docherty, PhD, ATC, FNATA; Michael G. Dolan, MA, ATC; J. Ty Hopkins, PhD, ATC, FNATA; Eric Nussbaum, MEd, ATC; Wendy Poppy, MS, PT, ATC; Doug Richie, DPM, 'National Athletic Trainers' Association Position Statement: Conservative Management and Prevention of Ankle Sprains in Athletes': https://meridian.allenpress.com/jat/article/48/4/528/191258/National-Athletic-Trainers-Association-Position

p. 192 Robert W Morton, Kevin T Murphy, Sean R McKellar, Brad J Schoenfeld, Menno Henselmans, Eric Helms, Alan A Aragon, Michaela C Devries, Laura Banfield, James W Krieger, Stuart M Phillips, 'A systematic review, meta-analysis and meta-regression of the effect of protein supplementation on resistance training-induced gains in muscle mass and strength in healthy adults': https://bjsm.bmj.com/content/52/6/376.full?fbclid=IwAR2nbGAY0FFJAcdwl_cdiv6uaNGHMpQ9rLSNb7xrWfigtoR3T30MzTok2P4

pp. 206–208 J S Volek , N D Duncan, S A Mazzetti, R S Staron, M Putukian, A L Gómez, D R Pearson, W J Fink, W J Kraemer, 'Performance and muscle fiber adaptations to creatine supplementation and heavy resistance training': https://pubmed.ncbi.nlm.nih.gov/10449017/

pp. 217–218 BMI Healthcare.co.uk, 'Men and mental health: a damaging stigma':https://www.bmihealthcare.co.uk/health-matters/mens-health/men-and-mental-health-a-damaging-stigma#gdpr-out

INDEX